Praise for *Dialectical Behavior Therapy for Wellness and Recovery: Interventions and Activities for Diverse Client Needs*

"It is exciting when a book comes along in the mental health field that both changes the way we think about our work and can be immediately applied to our work in a practical way, and Andrew Bein's book does just that! As a mindfulness-oriented therapist in a busy university counseling center, I am excited to start using this book in my work with clients, and I know it will be a resource I will turn to again and again."

Ronni Arensberg, PsyD, LP,
North Dakota State University Counseling Center

"Andrew Bein's latest book brilliantly captures the essence of DBT and integrates self-regulatory concepts that are key to healing trauma. The practical exercises and monitoring tools are excellently designed and will be helpful tools that will enhance recovery. This book will not only be useful for clinicians but clients as well."

Elaine Miller-Karas, LCSW; Executive Director
of the Trauma Resource Institute

"This is a thoughtful book that dares to venture into the uncharted territory of rethinking treatment for persons diagnosed with personality disorders based on the recovery paradigm. While DBT has always been a respectful, and empowering, approach, Bein courageously challenges some of the core assumptions upon which traditional psychotherapeutic practice has been based in order to engage clients in a more collaborative relationship that enables them to assume an active, and central, role in their own recovery."

Larry Davidson, PhD, Professor of Psychiatry,
Yale University School of Medicine

T0201228

"Like water on rock, Dr. Bein reshapes Dialectical Behavior Therapy with a deepened appreciation for emotion regulation through mindfulness practice. This practical and clearly presented model offers a much needed treatment model for use in diverse settings. It is filled with simple, well-constructed exercises and tools that make basic DBT principles more accessible than ever before. *Dialectical Behavior Therapy for Wellness and Recovery* is an invaluable contribution not only for therapy, but for quality everyday living."

Satsuki Ina, PhD, MFT; Director, Family Study Center; Producer and Director, *Children of the Camps*

"Dr. Bein skillfully brings DBT, essential mindfulness practices, and skills-building to the everyday world of therapists and clients. Andy presents a cohesive and comprehensive model of integrative therapy that benefits those willing to take on practices promoting growth and development from the ground up."

Edward Brown, Zen priest; Author; *Tassajara Bread Book*

"Dr. Bein's thoughtful exploration of recovery reminds us that our clients bring extraordinary strengths and life experience to the healing process. The book's concepts are presented in ways that are refreshing and new, giving the clinician immediate clarity and sense of how to teach the material. I plan to use DBT-WR for my next therapy group."

Nancy White, LCSW, Private Practice; Former DBT Group Leader, Kaiser Permanente

"Bein writes with authenticity and empathy, and, in his strong and soft voice, concepts such as intention, self-compassion, mindfulness, and radical acceptance become not only of therapeutic value but a template for all of us to live with presence and integrity."

Shauna L. Smith, MSW, LMFT; Author, *Making Peace With Your Adult Children: A Guide to Family Healing*; Co-Founder, Therapists for Social Responsibility

DIALECTICAL BEHAVIOR THERAPY FOR WELLNESS AND RECOVERY

INTERVENTIONS AND ACTIVITIES FOR DIVERSE CLIENT NEEDS

ANDREW BEIN

WILEY

Cover Image: ©iStockphoto.com/antishock
Cover design: Andrew Liefer

This book is printed on acid-free paper.♾

Published by John Wiley & Sons, Inc., Hoboken, New Jersey
Published simultaneously in Canada

For general information about our other products and services, please contact our Customer Care Department within the United States at (800) 762-2974, outside the United States at (317) 572-3993 or fax (317) 572-4002.

Wiley publishes in a variety of print and electronic formats and by print-on-demand. Some material included with standard print versions of this book may not be included in e-books or in print-on-demand. If this book refers to media such as a CD or DVD that is not included in the version you purchased, you may download this material at http://booksupport.wiley.com. For more information about Wiley products, visit www.wiley.com.

Library of Congress Cataloging-in-Publication Data

Bein, Andrew M.
    Dialectical behavior therapy for wellness and recovery : interventions and activities for diverse client needs /
    Andrew Bein.
        1 online resource.
    Includes bibliographical references and index.
    Description based on print version record and CIP data provided by publisher; resource not viewed.
    ISBN 978-1-118-65333-3 (pbk) — ISBN 978-1-118-69061-1 (ebk) — ISBN 978-1-118-75997-4 (ebk)
  1. Dialectical behavior therapy.   2. Mental health.   3. Clinical health psychology.   I. Title.
    RC489.B4
    616.89'142—dc23

                                                                                    2013021305

Printed in the United States of America

V10018447_050820

Contents

Foreword

Dialectical Behavior Therapy (DBT) was originated and developed by Dr. Marsha Linehan in the 1980s as a psychological intervention for persons with a history of multiple suicide attempts who were very sensitive to criticism and emotionally dysregulated. DBT combined principles and practices of behavior therapy with philosophies and therapeutic strategies designed to balance both acceptance of the client and efforts toward change in therapy simultaneously. The core elements of DBT, as described by Linehan and colleagues, include:

> (1) a biosocial theory of disorder that emphasizes transactions between biological disposition and learning; (2) a developmental framework of stages of treatment; (3) a hierarchical prioritizing of treatment targets within each stage; (4) delineation of the functions that treatment must serve, and treatment modes to fulfill those functions; and (5) sets of acceptance strategies, change strategies, and dialectical strategies. (Robins, Schmidt, & Linehan, 2004, pp. 31–32)

Dr. Andrew Bein, in this pioneering new book, has taken DBT to another level of innovation, in what he terms *dialectical behavior therapy for wellness and recovery* (DBT-WR). Dr. Bein's innovation, in this richly detailed and highly practical volume, is to develop a DBT-informed approach that draws from his extensive clinical practice experience, rigorous DBT training, and his own extensive training and practice in mindfulness meditation. DBT-WR, as so clearly described in this volume, has been developed so as to be appropriate for application in community mental health, private practice, residential day treatment, and high school settings, and particularly for persons having substance abuse histories and dual diagnoses.

Dr. Bein's approach in DBT-WR reflects not only his deep appreciation of relevant clinical science and his clinical practice experience, but also draws extensively from his own long-term meditation practice and review of recent neuroscientific studies of meditation, particularly mindfulness meditation.

Meditation has been attracting an increasing number of persons in recent years, witnessed by the number of books, magazines, and websites concerned with meditation. Various clinical interventions involving meditation practices have been taught within such contexts as hospitals, clinics, and schools. Over the past few decades, there has been a dramatically increasing number of published cognitive, affective, and neuroscientific studies of meditation practice and meditation-derived clinical interventions, and in the funding of such studies by governmental and private sources. Research within this growing domain, now being referred to as "contemplative science," has frequently focused on attention, memory, emotion response, and emotion regulation, in both long-term and short-term practitioners of meditation such as Buddhist and other spiritual traditions, as well as in those provided brief training in the modern secular form referred to as *mindfulness meditation*. The results of this body of research, as pointed out by Dr. Bein in this volume, have particular relevance for how he has conceptualized and applied DBT-WR in his clinical practice and training of students.

In light of these societal, scientific, and clinical/educational developments, Dr. Bein's new book seems particularly timely, filling a need for specific guidance being sought by clinicians who wish to bring the benefits of DBT- and mindfulness-informed therapies to a wide range of persons within mental health, substance abuse treatment, and educational settings. The clarity of Dr. Bein's writing further enhances both the practical value and pure pleasure of reading this important contribution. It is my hope that it will be widely read, positively influencing both present and future generations of practitioners.

Alfred W. Kaszniak, PhD
Professor of Psychology, Neurology,
and Psychiatry
University of Arizona

Preface

Nearly 25 years ago, Dr. Marsha Linehan forged a different way of working with clients combining traditions of Western psychology and Eastern thought. Her depth of wisdom and clarity of vision were compelling, as she fashioned the dialectical behavior therapy (DBT) approach. DBT addressed the change-acceptance paradox present in therapeutic endeavors and brilliantly integrated pragmatic and self-empowering skill-building for clients who were considered among some of the hardest to reach, those diagnosed with borderline personality disorder. The perfect storm of Dr. Linehan's emergent interest in and practice of mindfulness; her depth of understanding the clientele and ways the clientele could work effectively within the therapeutic process; her commitment to empirical research; her unconventional style; and her deep, heartfelt connection to those who were suffering contributed to what DBT is today. In recent years, Dr. Linehan has revealed her own emotional struggles, and we wonder to what degree her past challenges contributed to her profound wisdom and passion as well as DBT's evolution.

This book brings DBT to the different corners of the psychotherapy and counseling world—from the crisis residential program that usually works with clients from 1 to 3 months to the private practice office, where emotion regulation skills are on the plate along with other issues. It deals with the reality that, in many settings, people are either passing through quickly or experience barriers for traditional DBT engagement. Dr. Linehan developed her workbook based on clients who stayed in 2- to 3-hour DBT groups over the course of at least 1 year and had supplemental skills coaches (1993); present-day resources and support for therapy make these conditions rare.

Applying Dialectical Behavior Therapy

The approaches here are unique, pragmatic, and designed for the present-day realities of many mental health practitioners and their diverse clients. The model and activities capture the major principles of DBT; however, it is reconfigured enough to be a *DBT-informed practice*. The model and activities reflect my DBT training, mindfulness training, and direct practice and evaluation in the following settings: community mental health, substance abuse with women, dual diagnosis, private practice, high school mental health, and residential day treatment. The Chapter 6 lessons and activities have been used with groups and individuals, and the treatment approach integrates a wellness and recovery orientation, thus the treatment is referred to as *dialectical behavior therapy for wellness and recovery* (DBT-WR).

Competence With the Realities of Practice

The book's discussion of interventions, guiding framework, and its precise client activities respond to practice environment and practitioner realities and offer the following elements.

Access to DBT for Diverse Clientele   Transdiagnostic clients benefit from DBT-WR. They do not need to receive the whole, traditional DBT package in order to reduce their emotional reactivity, enhance the skillfulness of their responses, and learn how to live more effectively and joyfully in the here and now. Use of this book will help clients gain access to DBT interventions in a manner similar to the way clients, across populations and settings, benefit from cognitive behavior therapy interventions.

Practice Model That Facilitates Client Integration of DBT   A simplified model is more memorable for clients—especially shorter term ones. This model starts with the client intention to practice Wise Mind and then focuses on acceptance and improving the moment as core strategies in order to deal with difficulty. Client self-compassion supports the entire endeavor. The complete model is pictorially represented (see Chapter 6), which is helpful for more visual learners. (The practitioner version of the model is found in Chapter 2.) Easily comprehended neuroscience explanations are offered that motivate and interest clients. One finding discussed in the book was how much providing neuroscience information helped clients feel like they were being respected for their intelligence.

Clear Activities Designed for Client Engagement   Fifteen practice lessons are clearly laid out in Chapter 6. Each lesson has a theme and activities reengage concepts from prior lessons because (a) it is important for clients to see and experience interconnections, for example, how mindfulness and acceptance helps someone come to terms with arising judgments; and (b) people may join open groups and interjection of earlier presented concepts helps them get "up to speed." Suggestions are provided at the beginning of Chapter 6 on ways to implement the 15 lessons and permission is granted to practitioners to reproduce these materials for their clients or consumers.

Comprehensible, Applicable Tools for Clinicians   Practitioners, regardless of prior experience or training, understand the DBT-WR principles as presented. Relevant dialectical relationships (or paradoxes) are depicted and explained throughout. Although the book is describing theory and practices that are profound, meaningful, and effective, the language is direct and presumes no particular practitioner background with DBT or mindfulness. The mindfulness tools presented in the book yielded client benefit as per Kentucky Inventory of Mindfulness Scale scores (Richards & Sehr, 2011).

Respects Client Diversity, Aspirations, and Meaning Systems DBT-WR grapples with the increasing expectation that mental health practitioners are accountable to mental health recovery principles. The book deals with the dilemma of how to flatten the practitioner–client hierarchy and not have DBT-WR work embody top-down, expert–nonexpert dynamics or reinforce stigma. Exploring the recovery paradigm, accounting for client ethnic/racial and cultural diversity, determining the relevance and use of motivational interviewing to spur engagement, and examining DBT-WR through a mental health recovery lens are unique and vital contributions.

Incorporates Substance Abuse and Dual Diagnosis Issues The interface of clients struggling with emotion regulation challenges and substance abuse is addressed. The DBT tradition has language that is parallel to 12-step programs and clinicians can make useful connections and distinctions. The degree to which our clients have a dual diagnosis needs to be considered in DBT-WR and data is provided. This book helps clinicians understand similarities and differences regarding mental health and substance abuse recovery as well as their respective treatment implications.

Accounts for Trauma and Engages in Neuroscience Discussions With Clients The implications of trauma for those receiving DBT-WR treatment is discussed. Many clients considered to have emotion regulation challenges have a history of trauma. This book accounts for issues such as validating people's experiences without, necessarily, deeply processing them; attuning to and effectively addressing people's activation or understimulation levels within sessions; engaging in related practices to help people learn to become grounded (e.g., cognitive-behavioral therapy and Trauma Resilience Model); and incorporating hopeful neuroscience discussions regarding neuroplasticity as well as fight–freeze–flight terminology for people struggling with posttraumatic stress disorder or other trauma-related effects.

Inclusive Spiritual Approaches The DBT-WR model integrates bigger picture or spiritual practices that assist people's emotion regulation and overall sense of wellness. The charge is that it is irresponsible to not account for and address this main source of hope, meaning, comfort, and well-being (see Hodge, 2005, for overview). DBT-WR directly opens possibilities for people to seek support from their higher power for emotion regulation, or to explore ways in which moving beyond their "small self" may be liberating. For people who are disabled, unemployed, or underemployed, reframing their "job"—in such terms *as how they inspire the world through their courage and personal healing*—can be powerful and comforting in times of despair, uncertainty, or boredom. Bigger picture strategies are inclusive of people on the spirituality spectrum from formally religious to nonreligious, humanist. The interface with 12-step spirituality is consistently examined.

Practitioner Use-of-Self Finally, the practitioner's use-of-self is investigated in Chapter 5. Some clinicians who had taken prior DBT workshops claimed that they never quite understood DBT until they were exposed to the use-of-self material in this book. This information is in service of clients who deserve to have practitioners who meaningfully integrate DBT-WR rather than approach it as a set of techniques. The material in this chapter is also in service of DBT-WR practitioners who find that embodiment and integration of mindfulness and radical acceptance, as well as their capacity to manifest a strong back and soft front (Bein, 2008) in the middle of uncertainty bring immeasurable reward, growth, and competence.

May this book be of benefit to you and your clients!

One

Applying Dialectical Behavior Therapy: Toward Access for Diverse Client Needs

Gifts of Dialectical Behavior Therapy

The tools and lessons of dialectical behavior therapy (DBT) may be seen as gifts for taking care of the self. Instead of suffering with a mind hijacked (Goleman, 1995) by emotional reactivity, pervasive and troublesome thoughts, and mood states, DBT clients learn to effectively deal with, cope with, and embrace life and arising moment-to-moment experience. There are two elements of DBT—a dialectic orientation and mindfulness—that are revolutionary in terms of a therapeutic method. We will briefly address these elements here but will explore them in more detail later.

A dialectic orientation squarely addresses and integrates a fundamental paradox of engaging in therapy. It identifies that at the core of the therapeutic process is the dynamic relationship between acceptance/validation and change. Other therapeutic modalities may emphasize that validation is important within the practitioner–client partnership in order to lay the groundwork for the real work of the endeavor: change. In DBT, the real work is both acceptance/validation and change.

In general, clients become clients because either they or people in their environments believe that they are in need of change. Distress and anxiety may be profound; depression or mania may be debilitating and/or dangerous; anger or reactivity may be difficult to contain. Troublesome emotions lead to negative and destructive behavior that has painful consequences for the client and for persons with whom the client is somehow connected. Therapy becomes part of a change project directed toward the client so that her or his emotions may become less troublesome and the resultant behavior less destructive. Cognitive-behavioral therapy (CBT) is the strategy most often pursued to create this change.

CBT emphasizes changing the thoughts or beliefs— "cognitive distortions"—that are seen to be at the source of troubling emotions and their resultant behaviors. The traditional sequence is outlined as dysfunctional thought → emotion → behavior. The client's job is learning how thoughts contribute to feelings and behavior and then, sometimes in the midst of challenging circumstances, to examine underlying thoughts. When the thoughts or thought patterns are identified that lead to troublesome emotions and behaviors, the task is to convert the thought or thoughts to ones that are more health promoting. The client may be fairly successful examining, deconstructing, then replacing thoughts in a practitioner's office; the trick is to stop the thought → emotion → behavior chain outside the office and to insert alternative cognitions as life unfolds.

DBT emerged partly from the discovery that CBT could be experienced by clients as invalidating. Let us consider the example of a female client who is struggling with her partner's remark regarding her weight. There may be various cognitions that, depending on the actual circumstances and client cognitive patterns, could be inserted in order to mediate against the distress provoked by the insulting comment: "I have had recent compliments about how beautiful I am, so I have a lot of evidence that I am in fact beautiful"; "my weight is not important—it's what's inside that counts"; I don't have to meet Western, patriarchal standards of thinness, I am fine just the way I am"; "my partner's comments are really about his/her hangups, I don't need to personalize them"; or "this is one negative comment, I am creating my own distress because I am catastrophizing" (personalizing and catastrophizing are two examples of distorted cognitive patterns). These kinds of cognitive affirmations or attempts at replacing negative thinking may be effective. At times, however, the practitioner's suggestion of these approaches implies to the client that her suffering is superficial or self-induced and could easily be relieved if she "just got her head on straight." In fact, this kind of unintended message has a way of sometimes reinforcing or adding on to problems; "not only am I always feeling hurt and hyper about my weight, but I am stupid for feeling this way."

In this cycle of shame and pain, the person continues attempting to replace one thought for another. While at a party her insecurity is traced to the thought of "I am unattractive, and I will never find a partner" and is replaced with "I am attractive and desirable," or some other related cognitive strategy. As Linehan (2005) has remarked, this kind of cognitive dance may actually reinforce the power and impact of the negative thought. It is sometimes difficult to defeat negative thinking with thought replacement or self-admonishments to basically "not think this way." A client has told me that for years—with the guidance of one therapist or another—she has attempted to replace thoughts related to how much of a loser she was. Despite temporary reprieves, the strategy fundamentally did not work. She would, in essence, push the negative, self-defeating thought into the closet and bring in alternative thoughts to occupy its place, only to have negative thoughts consistently reemerge demanding their place in the center of her mind.

The Dialectic Orientation

As an alternative to the notion that "I am thinking the wrong way" or the orientation of beating back thoughts with other thoughts, DBT begins with the idea that the experience of acceptance/validation lays the groundwork for change, fuels change, and makes meaningful change more likely. Thoughts arise and we see them for what they are—thoughts. Mindfulness, as we will discuss later, gives us clarity as to the nature of thoughts. We begin to realize that thoughts come into consciousness in a manner over which we have little control. This reality is brought home during any attempt at doing a mindfulness exercise and focusing on our breath. Despite our intentions, the brain continues to do its job and secrete thoughts in the same way that the liver secretes bile. There is no being, or ego, or separate self—a person with name X—that has ultimate control over this process.

We begin to realize that thoughts are insubstantial: they arise, they disappear, they trigger other thoughts, and they change. We accept that thoughts are thoughts, and this acceptance creates space around them. We do as Rumi suggests, invite them in for tea (i.e., accept them) but not beyond. We do not have to believe thoughts, and we do not have to ruminate. It is the ruminating and belief in our thoughts as truths that give thoughts the appearance of having solidity or substance. In DBT, if we do start ruminating or we notice that we are paying a lot of attention to unhelpful thoughts, we accept that we are doing just that—ruminating and engaged in hurtful thinking—and we make a decision to take care of ourselves.

Radical Acceptance as a Basis for Change

Emotional states may also be the starting point and source of thoughts and thought patterns (see Goleman, 2004). One time I was at a convocation of master's students and none of the students approached me to investigate whether they would want, in the following academic year, to do a thesis or research project with me. While I was standing in a large room alone, other faculty members had students gathered near them. I started telling myself the story of how other faculty members knew the students; I did not because I did not teach first-year master's students that year. That story was my attempt at feeling okay. Then my story moved to how economical and thoughtful I had been presenting my research interests at this meeting. Other narcissistic and less time-conscious faculty successfully self-promoted themselves, and now they were reaping the rewards of their efforts. During the next faculty meeting, I thought self-righteously, I will bring up how we need to have a short time limit to discuss our research interests so that the gathering does not last so long. I alternated between my thoughts about not knowing the students as the justification for their limited interest in making contact with me, and the thoughts about my higher level of consideration—relative to other faculty members—in an attempt to deal with my discomfort. I took a deep breath and allowed myself to notice the underlying emotion related to standing alone at this gathering. *I was feeling insecure.* From this place of insecurity or vulnerability I had launched into thoughts and stories that were actually enhancing my suffering and doing little to assuage my insecurity. I accepted or, as we will discuss later, *radically* accepted my insecurity. There was nothing more to do. Acceptance teaches us that we can hold these emotional states as they are. In this case, that was where the relief was located. I lightheartedly acknowledged and accepted that I had been all bound up in a story of excuses and self-righteousness because that's what humans do—make desperate, reactive attempts at feeling okay. In the end, I *regulated my emotions* through radically accepting all of it: the insecurity, the small me that was making up stories, the comparing mind that noticed who had more or fewer students near them.

From this place of acceptance, change occurs. We develop confidence that we have the ability to *respond* to life as it is and feel a sense of peace (or maybe just get a glimpse of peace) about thoughts, emotional states, and situations as they arise. Even if we are highly agitated or distressed, we cultivate the capacity to accept that we are agitated or distressed. Acceptance fuels a sense of compassion for ourselves and others. We become open to change, not so much because we are ashamed of ourselves or because we want other people to "get off our case" about changing, but *because we want to take care of ourselves*. We let go of some of the debilitating judgments and stories that we have about who we are, and realize that the best we can do is to respond today to live in a manner that is healthy and life promoting.

The *practitioner's* internalization and practice of acceptance for one's self as well as her acceptance of the client translate to how successfully the client will learn acceptance. (We will discuss ways in which the clinician's presence and personal work with radical acceptance can be developed.) We, as therapists or clinicians, can preach to our clients about acceptance or behave as if it is an elusive, mysterious state to be grasped and attained, or we can create a container in which the client experiences that she or he is radically accepted. This container is a base from which the client may begin to experience acceptance of her own thoughts, feelings, and responses. In an environment of acceptance there is less need to run from or avoid what is happening internally and less need to dress up, deny, or create a stir in order to hide one's internal life. The client senses that acceptance is available now, in this present moment. From this place of safety and from the enhanced capacity to face things as they are, change unfolds.

As we explore further in the book, we will see that mindfulness and acceptance are at the heart of emotion regulation and wellness. They slow down the reactive cycle and open possibilities for us to function in a manner that is calmer, less impulsive, more skillful, and less anxiety ridden.

The Relationship of Mindfulness and Acceptance

Mindfulness has a mutually reinforcing relationship with radical acceptance. When we are mindful, we attune to things as they are and begin to see clearly. The most fundamental mindfulness skill is to observe and describe phenomena without adding a

story or judgment to the description. This serves us in noticing, for example, the difference between thoughts and truths.
Noticing that I am having a thought that I am incompetent is
quite different from *fusing* with—that is, completely believing—
I am incompetent (Hayes & Lillis, 2012). Mindfulness allows us
to observe our emotional process and see, for example, the anger
arising. We learn from mindfulness exercises that our breath can
ground us and that the emotion of anger is not permanent and
not as solid as we may imagine. We see anger for what it is: a
passing emotional state, rooted in the body, that may be transformed through acceptance of its existence, a mindful return
to the breath, and pursuit of a skillful response. Mindfulness
allows us to see through the times when we believe that the narrative chatter or commentary about our lives is our actual life.
We learn that we have choices about this kind of monologue,
and we cultivate the capacity to return to the present moment.
The framework and activities described in this book have sta-
tistically significant evidence supporting efficacy for enhancing
client mindfulness, particularly with respect to the mindfulness component "acceptance without judgment" ($p < .001$)
(Richards & Sehr, 2011).

In the preceding example, acceptance of my insecurity
related to my capacity to be mindful. I could have continued on a path of reactivity and launched into a scathing mass
e-mail directed at my colleagues about how they needed to be
more sensitive about time parameters at major student–faculty
gatherings. I could have become angry enough that I stormed
out of the meeting or given off such a venomous vibe that no
students would have wanted to approach me. (Some students
did end up speaking with me; perhaps they were feeling sorry
for me.) I could have internalized the distress and not acted
out, instead feeling depressed and alienated about the event.
With that alienated emotional state as a base, I may have built
a mental monument about how superior I was relative to
others. Being mindful of my distress, however, allowed me

to tune into what was occurring. I was able to see that my thoughts about myself and others were just thoughts and judgments and were not truths. I did not feel bad or ashamed at myself for having these thoughts. Then I sensed that insecurity—the best name I could come up with—was at the source of my distress. Accepting this process, allowed me to see and "stay with" the insecurity. Being mindful of things as they were was part of my acceptance of things as they were.

DBT was originally developed for people diagnosed with borderline personality disorder. Linehan's vision to adopt mindfulness as a core skill was to help clients not get lost in reactivity, to attune—in the moment—to the nature of distress, and to provide opportunities for skillful response. Additionally, mindfulness is about engagement in the present moment, as she has described, throwing yourself into life, getting up to bat and hitting the fastballs that life keeps throwing at you (Linehan, 2005). Thoughts and feelings arise; they are to be seen, acknowledged, and accepted. Then our task is to come back to the *present moment* of our life where the situation is nearly always workable and freedom is possible. Our return to the breath in a mindfulness exercise is our return to this present moment and is a metaphor and practice opportunity for living a fulfilling life.

Dialectical Behavior Therapy for Wellness and Recovery (DBT-WR)

Some 20 years ago Marsha Linehan (1993) and dialectical behavior therapy (DBT) reached prominence. At the time, the treatment primarily targeted people suffering with borderline personality disorder and offered hope and real life results for many people who had previously been unresponsive to treatment. Linehan's commitment to the empirical validation of DBT, mounting evidence of DBT effectiveness, and practitioner thirst and enthusiasm for mindfulness-based approaches has meant the proliferation of DBT practice in all kinds of clinical contexts and situations.

Unfortunately, emergent DBT practice is often loosely conceptualized, and clients seem destined to take away fragmented chunks of DBT that may or may not produce compelling experiences, lessons, and skill mastery. While Linehan's clients "generally stay(ed) in psychosocial skills training for at least 1 year" (Linehan, 1993, p. 11) and had therapists as well as "skills trainers," present practice realities seldom afford these kinds of client and practitioner resource opportunities and thus demand systematic thinking for making DBT application relevant.

The empirically supported DBT-informed practice approach offered here – *hereinafter referred to as DBT for wellness and recovery, or DBT-WR* – will address important client and service context realities and the questions and concerns that emanate from them.

➤ Clients may be exposed to a limited number of DBT groups or individual sessions. Crisis residential programs, in-patient hospital-based programs, intensive outpatient programs, and cycles within the calendars of community mental health agencies mean that clients receive something called DBT, but may be getting 5, 8, or 12 sessions. One ultra-prestigious psychiatric hospital, for example, has patients cycling in and out of the in-patient "DBT groups," and, whether they are diagnosed with schizophrenia or depression, haphazardly working through Linehan's (1993) manual. How can there be enough integrity to these kinds of experiences for them to be meaningful?

➤ Clients involved in some form of DBT practice have variant capacities for holding concepts in their day-to-day consciousness. Instead of multiple, abstract concepts and approaches helping the client to live, in Linehan's words, a life worth living, can there be a simple unifying approach that a client can call upon and remember in daily life and in the midst of emotional distress?

➤ Some DBT clients have disdain for "homework," and there are psychological barriers (e.g., past school failure), cognitive challenges, limited literacy, and compromised environments (e.g., lack of home, chaotic families, or exhausting lives) that make doing homework improbable. In one ongoing DBT-WR group I conducted, group work was part of a women's perinatal drug treatment program, which demanded individual work, 12-step attendance, weekly meetings with a sponsor, abstinence, maintenance of a constructive relationship with their Child Protective Services worker, individual therapy, daily 3-hour involvement with their peers, parenting skills training, and practical and/or emotional resolution of their trauma. These demands were over and above either ongoing child rearing of sometimes challenging children or regular supervised parent–child visits for children that were in foster care arrangements. Insisting on homework completion for these women would have been unreasonable and invalidating. How can we be responsive to the varying degrees to which homework completion makes sense?

➤ Mental health agencies increasingly embrace mental health recovery as the dominant framework for delivering services (see Slade, 2009; Walsh, 2013). Within this paradigm, we are admonished to tune into the aspirations of our clients, maintain a collaborative, nonexpert stance, celebrate gains, and move beyond traditional clinical boundaries that may be overly detached and impersonal. What kind of language can we use within DBT-WR applications that is more inviting and less triggering, and that flattens the hierarchy? How can the DBT-WR process solicit and incorporate client solutions, wisdom, and worldview rather than reproducing hierarchy and disempowerment through notions of depositing skills and expert knowledge?

➤ Client spirituality is increasingly seen as a significant force in client wellness and recovery. Not accounting for spirituality is argued to be clinically irresponsible (Hodge, 2005; Bein, 2008). How can DBT-WR incorporate spirituality in an inclusive manner so that it may serve as an ongoing resource for emotion regulation and wellness?

➤ Mindfulness activities produce a variety of responses. Some people are encouraged with the possibilities while others are agitated with their sense of being inadequate mindfulness failures. Some people are suspicious that mindfulness interferes in some way with their religious traditions; others experience mindfulness as invoking an open field where invasive and frightening experiences may arise unimpeded. How can we approach mindfulness so as to reduce the client's familiar and discouraging thoughts related to performance and success or failure? How can we adapt mindfulness work to be inclusive of unique client needs and cultural belief systems, and what kind of clinician mindfulness practice is advisable in order to facilitate client progress?

➤ Skills training may normalize struggle and challenge, and the acquisition of DBT-WR skills may facilitate a sense of mastery, competence, and stability. However, the very process of teaching already disempowered clients how to think, feel, and behave may be experienced as denigrating. One memorable Latina DBT client once asked me in a nonaccusatory tone, "Are you trying to teach us to behave more like White people?" Teaching skills in mandated settings may invoke ambivalent feelings; however, one finding from recent DBT-WR groups was that clients deeply appreciated being taught neuroscience. Not only did simple neuroscience explanations validate the emotional difficulties clients had faced as a result of trauma, but clients also reported that neuroscience discussions and being shown a model of the brain indicated respect for their intelligence (Richards & Sehr, 2011). How may we bring the riches of neuroscience into DBT in a way that (a) validates client struggles with emotion regulation, (b) enhances their enthusiasm for and belief in emotion regulation, and (c) clarifies and opens a window to the possibilities for developing an effective and balanced mind—referred to as Wise Mind?

➤ Client radical acceptance is a skill, is a goal, and ultimately is intimately connected to mindfulness practice. Clients cultivate the capacity for radical acceptance through the didactic presentation of related skills and activities, and through their internalized experience of the practitioner's radical acceptance of them. How do we manifest, with challenging clients, a sense that we completely embrace them for who they are? How far-reaching is radical acceptance and what use-of-self orientations help us regulate boundaries and our emotional life as we interact with our clients?

➤ DBT founder Marsha Linehan asserts that practitioners present "unrelenting insistence on total abstinence" (Denning & Little, 2012). However, various service contexts providing DBT emphasize harm reduction. HIV-oriented programs, for example, may work with people to collaboratively evaluate the degree to which drug and alcohol use is either a threat to safety or is in some manner a resource helping the individual cope with trauma (Denning & Little, 2012). Other settings such as housing-first residences, community mental health programs, and universities are mandated to work with and not exclude clients who engage in varying degrees of harmful behavior. Embedded in this work are motivational interviewing approaches that may, in fact, enhance the degree to which clients experience radical acceptance. What kinds of DBT-WR adaptations can be made at agencies where the leadership and staff value motivational interviewing and will not insist on certain behavior in order to qualify for service? What may be the strengths and weaknesses, as it applies to the implementation of DBT, of this more permissive environment?

➤ Finally, the historical development of DBT proceeded on the foundation that creating change in the lives of desperate, emotionally dysregulated, and—in traditional clinical terms— highly resistant clients demanded clear boundaries and, as Shulman (1999) would say, a "demand for work." One manifestation of this orientation is the four-absence limit (Reynolds, Wolbert, Abney-Cunningham, & Patterson, 2007) that clients may not exceed in order for them to remain in a DBT program. At one community mental health clinic, I observed a fairly talented clinician recruit clients and run a group with these attendance parameters. At the end of 6 months, her DBT "group" had a total of one client who completed treatment. In the name of treatment fidelity, the rigid adherence to attendance parameters, in essence, helped establish conditions for "creaming" the population down to one successful client. The inadvertent institutional contribution to creating drop-outs or push-outs meant that many community clients were left underserved. While observing this experience unfold, I radically accepted my sadness and decided on the skillful response of developing a pragmatic, responsive alternative to DBT delivery. Clients who have resource challenges—transportation issues, subsistence income, child care demands, waxing and waning energy or commitment to therapy, mental illness symptomology, medication problems, family crises, struggles with personal organization, and limited funding for formalized services—should be able to access the benefits of DBT even though they cannot participate in traditional delivery. In addition, agencies or settings that have shoestring or barely existent training budgets, crushing clinician or medical provider productivity demands, limited time for consultation and supervision, and practitioners playing multiple roles with clients should be able to offer clients the benefits of DBT. This book presents dialectical behavior therapy for wellness and recovery (DBT-WR), founded upon practice experience and supportive evidence. It is presented in the spirit of inclusivity, access, and pragmatism.

Two

Emotion Regulation and Resilience: Developing Wise Mind

Emotions are viewed as body-oriented responses to stimuli. Emotions prepare us to meet an arising situation and mobilize and direct our action. They engage whole-body phenomena in terms of our subjective experience, physiology, and behavior (Mauss, Levenson, McCarter, Wilhelm, & Gross, 2005). Other affective processes—mood, impulses, and stress—are conceptually distinguished from emotion. Moods are viewed as longer lasting and more diffuse than emotions and as having a less direct connection to specific situations or events. Impulses are distinguished from emotions in that they are less flexible and have a narrower range of behavioral targets. Impulses motivate approach-avoidance thoughts and actions regarding objects of pleasure and pain (Gross, 2007, as cited in Richards & Sehr, 2011). Finally, stress is seen as a negative response to challenging and taxing circumstances, while emotions have a more substantial range and may be experienced as either positive or negative (Gross & Thompson, 2007).

Emotion regulation efforts incorporate all of these elements, and the goal is to change core affect (Koole, 2009). The building thermostat is used as a metaphor to depict regulation. When the air is cold in the dwelling, the thermostat registers that fact and prompts the furnace to click on and keep the environment warm and relatively comfortable. When the dwelling is heated (or cooled) adequately—in other words, when a basic level of comfort or equilibrium is attained—the thermostat turns off the system. A functioning thermostat continues to regulate the temperature of the building and will do what is necessary to maintain the desired temperature range. A person who is dys-regulated has a thermostat that is not working properly. The heat may be blasting even though the house is hot; the air con-ditioning may come on during cold weather. There is limited capacity to regulate one's self and keep the temperature within a predictable range. An experience of disappointment not only feels like intense heat, but there is limited capacity to bring the heat down or modulate the emotion. A person may feel fro-zen and immobilized in the whirling thoughts and emotions embedded in despair, but the person has limited facility to rebound and effectively respond.

When dysregulation is chronic, the person's emotional states may be reactive, rapidly fluctuating, and somewhat unpredictable. The capacity for self-soothing or returning to some sense of wellness may be compromised, and the per-son with emotion regulation challenges may engage in des-perate attempts to return to equilibrium. These attempts may take the form of substance use, self-harm, risky sexual activity, or engagement in idealized relationships (Fruzetti & Iverson, 2004). When life is desperate enough and relief from the per-petual roller coaster of emotional life—as well as from the dam-aging consequences that accrue from that life—does not seem possible, the contemplation of suicide may actually bring relief.

Emotion dysregulation is described as stemming from the following sources: (a) biological predisposition and vulnerabil-ity, (b) an invalidating social environment, and (c) the transac-tion between the two elements (Linehan, 1993). Regardless of whether emotional vulnerability originated predominantly in the person's predisposed biological makeup or originated in the invalidating experiences that compromised biological resilience, people who struggle with emotion regulation, in particular those diagnosed with borderline personality disorder, seem to be highly sensitive to different life situations that arise. In addition to emotional sensitivity, the person's capacity for modulating strong emotions or returning to baseline before engaging in emotion-fueled actions is compromised (Linehan, 1993). In the case of some highly reactive people, it may be challenging to ascertain an actual "emotional baseline."

In the dialectical behavior therapy for wellness and recovery model (DBT-WR) presented in this book, there are three major strategies for effectively addressing emotional regulation challenges: (a) mindfulness of the moment, (b) responding to the moment, and (c) expanding the moment. An overview of these strategies will be presented. There are two elements that support these strategies and overall emotion regulation: the client's *intention to practice Wise Mind* and her/his cultivation of *self-compassion*. After these discussions, the issue of validation will be explored. Not only is there a focus on client self-compassion so that she or he may feel supported and patiently guided from within, the practitioner's responsibility is to stay vigilant about creating a validating helping environment. Finally, the model emphasizes that the person who is engaged in one or more strategies for regulating arising in-the-moment emotions or who is engaged in building emotional resilience is "residing" in their Wise Mind. *The terminology of Wise Mind serves as a landing point and constant reminder for people who wish to experience a sense of wellness and a reduced propensity for emotional reactivity.*

Emotion Regulation Strategies and Helping Framework

In DBT-WR, mindfulness helps regulate the thermostat and positively contributes to each of the emotion regulation areas discussed above. Mindfulness creates opportunities for choice between an arising situation and our response. Developing skill in mindfulness means that we have enhanced capacity to observe our anticipatory thoughts and feelings about situations, observe our internal life as we interact in various contexts and with people, and notice responses as they begin to arise or as they actually manifest themselves. This *observing stance* means that we are less likely to be caught in a blinding reactive cycle and less likely, as mentioned before, to *fuse* with this cycle.

Fusing with various emotional states or with particular thoughts means that we lose perspective regarding their pervasiveness and solidity. In the midst of anger or fear or despair about a particular situation, we may feel as if these emotions have taken over our life. Without being aware, our entire thought process may become fixated with a troubling situation. Fusing perpetuates the cycle of negative thinking and painful emotions. As thinking and emotion reinforce one another, sometimes exerting pressure downward, our behaviors reflect this fusion process. Thus, if we are feeling slighted and our emotional response is anger and distress, we may decide to act out our anger and, for example, text a nasty message to a person we feel has harmed us. This behavior, in fact, unskillfully fuses us further with the thoughts and emotions around betrayal, victimization, and unsatisfying relationships. We may add to the story and become convinced that these emotions will not go away, that positive relationships are not to be had, and that life will stay dreary.

We continue to develop unskillful strategies (Strosahl & Robinson, 2008) that reflect our cognitive and emotional states. We decide to not socialize and to sleep long hours in order to not have to deal with the possible conflicts that future social interactions may entail. We decide to run away from our emotions with long sessions of television watching or mindless time on the Internet. We also come to believe that we will cope with difficult situations through numbing ourselves with drugs and alcohol.

The Unskillful Response of Autopilot and Skillful Alternatives

Living on autopilot refers to a life lived unconsciously or guided by a set of conventions or expectations that are rarely examined (Strosahl & Robinson, 2008). In this autopilot-dominated life: (a) we are not mindful of our intentions, (b) we take circumstances for granted, (c) we are barely aware of our surroundings and our behavior as we move through the day, and (d) we default to "automatic" behavioral patterns when we encounter particular kinds of situations. Autopilot living indicates a life in which we go through the motions; it leaves us susceptible to emotional reactivity and nonmindful responses. We present the difficulties of autopilot to provide clients tools and perspectives for living a life worth living. The goal of work is always in service to client interests rather than to teach them how to be well behaved or to be "good clients."

This orientation to mental health wellness practice leads us to utilizing the word *skillful* rather than the commonly used term *appropriate*. The word *appropriate* often orients clients toward conforming to the rules and expectations of the institutional structure that holds power over them. Lecturing to clients about whether their behavior was appropriate does not help them deeply address emotion regulation challenges. Yes, many times it is helpful to learn about the expectations and limits within the social environment; however, labeling behavior as *inappropriate* may reinforce for the client that (a) the practitioner's job is to turn the client into a better-behaved individual; (b) the practitioner is the moral arbiter of the client's behavior; or (c) the process of examining and working on topics such as emotional reactivity or substance abuse is slanted toward the client making a *moral* choice that the clinician would approve of rather than toward the client's aspirations for wellness and recovery.

When we orient ourselves to client skillfulness, we examine the degree to which client behavior, effort, and intention are directed toward meeting her goals for wellness. If the client wants to have decent relationships and does not want to have intensely conflictual and emotionally draining interactions, we can reflect with him or her about a recent situation where she "cursed out" an acquaintance. As we collaboratively examine the events, the client may take the lead in proclaiming that her approach was not helpful for where she wants to go in her life (i.e., it was unskillful). If, as clinician, I instead proclaimed that cursing out an acquaintance was inappropriate, I slip into the pitfalls suggested earlier and reinforce the disempowering elements of the expert–nonexpert dichotomy.

There are five ways in which we may *skillfully* address autopilot tendencies, regulate emotions, and enhance wellness. Providing fuel for the implementation and effectiveness of each approach is adopting the intention to be in Wise Mind. That intention keeps us on the path of mindful interaction with ourselves and the world and assists us to respond and engage in health-promoting ways. All the DBT-WR approaches involve being **mindful of the moment**—which means *observe* what is happening internally, *describe* it, and *radically accept* it—as the starting point. From this base of mindfulness, there are different ways that we can **respond to the moment**. First, we can respond to the moment by *letting go*, which means releasing some emotional charge and intensity and being in the flow with things as they are. Second, we may respond to the moment by utilizing the skillful response of *self-soothing*. The third category of responses emphasizes engagement with *positive activities*, and the fourth approach includes the response strategy *opposite action*. The fifth approach entails **expanding the moment** or embracing a spiritual view. Some may appreciate the language of moving beyond "the small self" or connecting to the "bigger picture." *Expanding the moment* may be the primary response to mindful awareness of the moment or it may be in conjunction with other skillful responses (see Figure 2.1, p. 23).

Just as **intention** fuels our engagement with the overall effort to be in Wise Mind and to engage in one of the five approaches mentioned, **self-compassion** encourages us along the way to keep up the good fight. We will continue to struggle and trip up; self-compassion allows us to be radically accepting of our troubles and cheers us on, reminding us that we are worth caring about.

In the subsequent sections, we will gain understanding of these concepts and see how they interact in DBT-WR. Client lessons and activities in Chapter 6 correspond to the issues discussed.

The Skillfulness of Intention: Am I in Wise Mind?

When we are mindful of our intentions, we have the chance to have our highest aspirations and values guide our behavior. We take a moment and tap into a part of ourselves that may want to show up with energy and integrity instead of, for example, trying to take the easy way out. We might realize, as we contemplate cursing someone out, that our intentions are hidden from ourselves. When we are honest and mindfully assess the situation, we realize that the feelings that the other may experience as a result of our behavior are not on our radar, and that, in fact, cursing out the other person comes from our intention to get revenge. We make a decision about whether we wish to have our behavior reflect this previously obscured intention or whether we wish to cultivate an intention of invoking kindness and repairing our relationship.

Examining intentions can create changes in the way you, as the practitioner, approach the client's therapy experience. Does the client's form of participation relate to her or his desire to be liked, to appear cute, to make sure the therapist does not get too intimate, or to go through the motions because the service is mandated.

Instead of implicit intentions or reactive emotionality driving the bus, we and our clients have the chance to take the wheel and make our intentions explicit and conscious. When intentions are made explicit, we may transform our habitual way of doing things. Imagine what it would be like for people to:

> Show up to an activity with the intention to get the most out of it and to put forth significant effort.

> Have the intention to focus on the positives of a person and to let go of judgments.

> Walk outside with the intention to truly see the natural world, even in the most urban environment.

> Have the intention to not have problems define the day and to connect to the bigger, spiritual view (discussed later).

> Carry the intention of not provoking conflict with others.

> Have the intention of engaging in wellness-related activities.

> Hold the intention of not letting certain circumstances bring you down.

> Maintain the intention of living in Wise Mind in a state of emotional wellness.

The Intention to Practice Wise Mind

Being in Wise Mind incorporates the above intentions as well as the intention to practice the skills of mindfulness of the moment, responding to the moment, and expanding the moment. The intention to practice Wise Mind means to direct efforts at taking care of ourselves and our well-being. Taking care of ourselves essentially means taking care of the moment. We maintain the commitment to be mindful of whatever unfolds and to engage or respond skillfully.

In consulting Figure 2.1, the question "Am I in Wise Mind?" guides the intention for emotional regulation. The

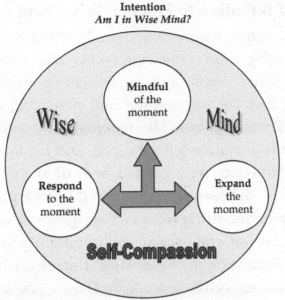

Primary Activities

Mindful: *Accept* the moment, *observe and notice* in the moment, and *be* in the moment.

Respond: *Improve* the moment and *let go* of the emotional charge of the moment, *be response-able* in the moment—*self-soothe, engage in positive actions, do opposite action.*

Expand: *Find meaning* in the moment and *connect to bigger picture*, love, or spirituality in the moment.

Figure 2.1   **Overview of Wise Mind**

question invites exploration into how much we (or the client) are *aligned with the intention* to move out of autopilot and practice in such a manner that furthers capacity for and experience of emotional regulation and mental wellness. The spirit of invitation embedded in a question is congruent with a motivational interviewing orientation (as we will discuss later), and provides an individual an idiosyncratic entry point into Wise Mind practice. "I don't know . . . am I in Wise Mind?"; "Oh yeah, I guess I'm not in Wise Mind . . . I kind of forgot"; "I feel like I was in Wise Mind, but now I got thrown off"; "Oh yeah, I need to take care of myself with Wise Mind, what a good reminder"; "I feel like I've been on autopilot and need to chill out . . . maybe I'll try that Wise Mind crap"; or as one clinical supervisee reflected, "I like the idea of Wise Ass more than Wise Mind." Wise Mind incorporates not only the skill components of relating to the moment through mindfulness, responding, and expansion; there is also an ease or a spirit of "I am being me right now, and that is okay."

Application of Intention to Practice Wise Mind

Intention is sometimes the missing ingredient between under-standing, digesting, and practicing skills and consistently remembering, calling upon, and implementing the skills. In one instance, I had been presenting and practicing DBT-WR skills with a 17-year-old boy. His parents had reported that prior efforts with therapists left him cold, and his interactions with these practitioners were limited and, ultimately, unsuc-cessful. The DBT-WR lessons presented in this book provided a launching point for discussing various challenges with emotional regulation, and he was enthusiastic about mindfulness and the potential of incorporating the Wise Mind framework. He even practiced mindfulness between sessions. During one session he reported how difficult it had been to sleep the night before; he was now quite tired. We talked about ways of applying mindfulness in situations like this one. I self-disclosed, encouraged to some degree within DBT (Koerner, 2012), about my own sleep adven-tures and ways of regulating emotions during challenging eve-nings. When I am awake during the night, I told him, I let go of stories about how long I have been awake and how many times I have awakened, as well as anticipatory stories regarding how my mood or energy will be affected in the morning from broken or limited sleep. In that manner, all that is happening moment to moment is my state of being in that moment. Each moment is fine as it is. Suffering enters a given moment when I plug into some kind of narrative about what is happening vis-à-vis my sleep. My intention is to be present in the moment, do what I need to do for myself to take care of my needs—which involves, at times, attending to asthma related effects—and to return to the bed and the breath. Each mindful breath is an opportunity for relaxation and sets the ground for sleepiness and a sleep state "to enter." There is no story about how long I have been lying in bed waiting to sleep and no story about how much lon-ger I will likely lie there. If worry thoughts enter such as "I need to fall asleep soon or else . . ." or evaluation thoughts enter such as "what a crappy night's sleep I am getting," returning to the breath allows evaluations, worries, or stories about time frames to drop off. The client was interested and declared his intention to apply the elements that were discussed.

We investigated what that prior night looked like for him, and he reported that throughout the night he was hot, and the room was stuffy. He continually woke up during the night, then spent more than the usual amount of time trying to fall asleep, amidst the discomfort. Although he knew about Wise Mind and the possibilities of responding to his emotional distress, he had not developed the intention—as borrowed from 12-step language—"to practice this way in all of his affairs." Had the intention to cultivate Wise Mind and maintain wellness been present, he would have been more likely to skillfully notice and radically accept what was happening (mindfulness) and respond to the situation by opening his room's window and allowing some cool, refreshing air to enter. Instead of this sequence, he was fused with both the distress about not sleeping and the worries and stories that seemed to inevitably flow. Wise Mind had been available all along, but could not be accessed in the middle of this distressing evening.

The relationship between intention and the practice of Wise Mind skills is dialectically related. A solidly held intention for emotional wellness serves as a reminder that all kinds of situations are ground for practicing Wise Mind. As situations arise, our intention inserts itself and manifests in the practice of skillful responses—thoughts, emotions, and behavior. Intention guides us toward skillful behavior rather than internalized admonitions of what we "should" do couched in the language of what is "appropriate." If we retrospectively reflect on the degree to which we utilized Wise Mind in response to a challenging situation, we do so within the framework of personal intentions, not shoulds and appropriateness.

How is intention regarding wellness generated and maintained? It emerges from the continued practice of Wise Mind skills. Practice, continued engagement, and repeated, sustained focus on the particular activities related to one's overall intention solidify and strengthen the intention itself. We may have the intention to play an instrument, eat well, or engage in some form of self-care; these intentions will be sustained with consistent behavior and practice that reflects the intention. However when we adopt an intention to eat a more healthy diet, our intention loses its foothold and becomes more like a resolution when our practice involves eating that is not mindful and instead defaults to familiar, unhealthy eating habits. The practice of mindfulness touches upon intentions and skillful practice. We stay aware of our intentions and this awareness helps drive the practices that will reinforce our intentions.

Resolutions as Distinct From Intention

The way that resolutions are conceptualized seems to have another quality. We do not connect to resolutions in the same manner. They are statements of behavioral change or they set a behavioral bar that we strive to attain. Buddhist psychology's critique of striving is that it is achievement and ego oriented. Thus, we become meritorious or worthy of praise or esteem when we have attained some external goal related to our resolution. The striving inherent in a resolution (such as a New Year's resolution) involves the separation between the ego-oriented concept of "I" and the behavior or achievement that "I" will attain. This kind of striving is embedded with judgments and evaluations of how well "I" am doing, and whether "I" deserve praise or blame based on the execution of the plan or the fulfillment of the resolution. Striving, then, places personal wellness in the hands of whether or not particular outcomes are attained. This approach is fraught with difficulties because (a) this external motivation strategy often does not work and resolutions are broken; (b) it reinforces a person's sense and internalized belief that the present moment is not the location of peace and wellness; (c) it creates personal pressure and places stress on someone to attain a particular outcome; (d) it reinforces a sense of personal failure when a resolution is not achieved; (e) it is embedded with the invalidating aspect that one's worthiness—or some would extend this further to say one's worthiness to be loved—is *contingent* on resolution fulfillment; (f) it does not account for the degree to which attainment or nonattainment is often a product of conditions that are beyond our control, thus implicitly endorsing the notion that personal will "conquers all."

The Intention of Self-Compassion

As you can see in Figure 2.1, self-compassion is the element that supports emotion regulation and Wise Mind work. Self-compassion serves as a protective factor against becoming dysregulated and enhances a sense of personal well-being. It quiets an inevitably critical voice and soothes us as we struggle with changing our familiar ways. Interestingly, as we move from autopilot to mindfully seeing things as they are, in other words with greater clarity, we may realize that some of our habitual patterns have caused harm not only to ourselves, but to others as well. As we fumble and bumble our way to living more in Wise Mind and less in emotional reactivity or self-harming behavior, our self-compassionate heart helps us be more patient with our struggles and setbacks and more forgiving and accepting of our failings and our limitations.

Kristin Neff (2011) states that self-compassion has three components:

First it requires *self-kindness*, that we be gentle and understanding with ourselves rather than harshly critical and judgmental. Second, it requires recognition of our *common humanity*, feeling connected with others in the experience of life rather than feeling isolated and alienated by our suffering. Third, it requires *mindfulness*—that we hold our experience in balanced awareness, rather than ignoring our pain or exaggerating it. (p. 42)

The cultivation of self-compassion occurs within the language of the 12 steps and is manifested in the way the meetings are conducted. Participants learn, particularly in the fourth step, that they have engaged in all kinds of acts and behaviors, yet as they read their fourth step or personal inventory to their sponsor and to their higher power, they sense they are still worthy of love. They also tend, during the meetings themselves, to love and care about the other struggling members of the fellowship. As people tell their stories of struggle and triumph, other attending members do not comment on what they have just heard. In that way the person who just spoke does not receive analysis, critique, feedback, or comparison from other members, just smiles, thank-yous, and occasional "keep coming back"s. The message is that no matter what you say or what you did, you are welcome here, without judgment. Newer participants begin to feel the quality of nonjudgmental acceptance of others and experience compassion for attendees as well as for their struggles. Over time, a newer member may experience that the quality of compassion is reciprocated in her direction; in other words, group members care about *you*, wish the best for *you*, and are willing to stand by *you*, regardless of your shameful story, to help you reduce your suffering and live a life worth living.

Compassion in this setting eventually comes around to self-compassion. First, you recognize that others are worthy of compassion and you begin to feel compassion for them. Second, you recognize that another's acceptance of you as well as their signs of support and caring for your struggles represents their compassion for you. Third, you begin to sense that there is compassion coming to you from something greater than yourself.

It may be from the love and compassion that is in the universe manifested in the beautiful beings in the 12-step rooms. It may be from a higher power and your higher power's or God's wish that you live well and feel loved. Finally, you feel compassion for yourself.

This vast container of compassion leads us to Neff's (2011) second component of self-compassion: a recognition of our common humanity. The power of the 12-step fellowship is to recognize that despite the degree to which you may have despised yourself for the kind of life you have led, you witness other human beings with the same kinds of struggles. You scratch below the surface and recognize the shared elements: pain, trauma, being lost and confused, acting tough to avoid feeling weak, numbing to not feel, having few places to turn, being betrayed by the ones who were supposed to care for you, struggling with whether to give up and return to the known life of drug use, the glimmer of hope and aspiration to live a life of integrity, and the personal exhilaration that comes from finally telling the truth. The beauty of 12-step work is that one's heart can crack open; movement toward feeling compassion for common humanity usually begins with everyone else. Eventually, compassion for one's self begins to take hold, and the shame that is integral to addiction recedes.

Group or individual DBT-WR practice mirrors these elements. In a group there is mutual witnessing of struggle and effort as people grapple with how and to what degree they will change their lives. People often cultivate nonjudgmentalism regarding other people's situations and efforts before they can treat themselves with similar kindness. The mental health practitioner or therapist in individual work creates a compassionate container where people's challenges, triumphs, and disappointments can be validated, normalized, and accepted. In addition to the process of establishing a favorable environment for facilitating self-compassion, there is explicit focus on building client self-compassion.

Mindfulness is Neff's (2011) final ingredient for self-compassion. Thus, in DBT-WR terms, mindfulness is dialectically related to self-compassion. Self-compassion helps us persist with Wise Mind practice in general, and mindfulness practice in particular, because we continue to trip up as we go along. Using a 12-step parallel, there is recognition that we will continue to make mistakes. In the tenth step, we are urged to continue taking personal inventory and to promptly admit to our wrongs. This is a mindful (and perhaps more critical) approach to maintaining awareness of what's going on in our minds and in our behavior. As we forget, get triggered, and lose our way, self-compassion provides a base encouraging us to return again and again, knowing that, just like so many others, we have bumps and setbacks along the road.

Mindfulness exercises such as short meditations are opportunities to practice the connection between mindfulness and self-compassion. We bring our mindful attention to our breath, and within a very short time we space out or move away from the breath. Eventually—although we may have drifted into the autopilot activity of getting lost in the narrative of our life—we click into the mindfulness skill of observing our process. We notice that attention has drifted from the breath, and we return to breath with self-compassion. If we instead return to the breath with a critical voice regarding how poorly we are doing, then mindfulness exercises become one more chance to be self-critical and denigrating. Even if we are self-critical, we can bring self-compassion to how self-critical we are. Eventually, the resting point becomes self-compassion.

There are a few more elements of self-compassion that should be clarified here. Compassion, unlike love, *specifically includes a wish and an aspiration to relieve suffering*. Thus, self-compassion hones in on the vulnerable, struggling person and wishes the best for that person. The compassionate heart is stirred by the efforts that are made in spite of adversity, by the mistakes that have been committed, and by the struggles and suffering that you, yourself, have had to endure. Self-compassion is intimately connected to these challenges and serves as an active cheerleader to encourage you to persevere in spite of them. "You are worth it," self-compassion says.

Self–Compassion and Radical Acceptance

Self-compassion reinforces the radical acceptance of self, thus it bolsters the primary dialectic in DBT-WR of acceptance and change. As mentioned, self-compassion directs the heart to encourage movement despite past or present thoughts, emotions, and behaviors. As we cultivate self-compassion, we are more comfortable with our distress and incline ourselves *to becoming our own ally*.

> If you can compassionately validate *your own* feelings, gently reminding yourself that it's only natural for you the feel the way you do . . . [y]ou can tell yourself what you really want to hear in the moment, "I'm so sorry you're feeling hurt and frustrated right now, what can I do to help?" (Neff, 2011, p. 228)

While being compassionate with one's self, you are less likely to spend time with and believe in the stories of the "comparing mind." This mind state frequently arises and contains messages regarding how we do not measure up to different people on a number of dimensions. You may tell yourself that others are superior to you in terms of appearance, intelligence, accomplishments, success of their children, or for having a better job, a better looking partner, more clean time, or a better sense of humor. Self-compassion diminishes the need for adopting a personal cognitive strategy of either reversing "who is better" (i.e., "she is not better than me; it is I who is superior") or the strategy of dismissing the importance of the comparison (i.e., "it really doesn't matter who is better"). Applying mindfulness to the comparing mind allows us to see the comparing mind for what it is—a normal generation of sto-ries—and then to make the decision not to dedicate attention to comparing mind's "noise." As comparing mind's influence recedes, we invite ourselves to feel self-compassion.

Part of our self-compassion involves mindfully being aware and *accepting* that comparing mind arises. In addition to apply-ing mindfulness, we see the universal nature of comparing mind and know that others suffer from comparing mind as well. Finally, we hold comparing mind with kindness. The ele-ments of mindfulness, universal nature, and kindness refer to Neff's (2011) three components. Engaging in this process pre-vents us from getting hooked, in other words from becoming reactive and emotionally dysregulated. We notice the tendency to be self-critical and self-judgmental, and we transform this tendency with an intention to be kind to ourselves and to not berate ourselves.

Externalizing Mind States and Self-Compassion Mind-fulness helps us see that mind states arise not governed by an omnipotent ego in control. Judgmental thoughts, angry incli-nations, and petty revenge fantasies may begin to arise or may take hold within our consciousness. Mind states here refer to the Eastern view of mind, which, literally translated from the Chinese character, is "heart–mind." In order to attain greater wellness and emotional regulation, we recognize and accept what is actually arising. We find ourselves within an interesting dialectic. Yes, it seems like these arising mind states are "yours." After all, they do not seem to "belong" to anyone else. In the convenience of language, we say "my anger," or "my thoughts about getting revenge"; yet, on the absolute level, there is really no ownership of these mind states. They are seen as rivers of emotion or thoughts that are universally shared and are not self-generated (Nhat Hanh, 1998). That is why the term *comparing mind* is used, making clear that it is not completely self-generated but is a universal mind state that may pass through consciousness.

Because of these dynamics, it makes sense to observe these arising phenomena without overidentifying particular thoughts and feelings as your own. In the end, you appreciate who you are, you value your resilience, you take care of yourself when you are vulnerable and in pain, and you provide comfort and refuge for yourself. Self-compassion helps you form an alliance with yourself as you embark on the difficult task of facing and taking responsibility where you can—your *response-ability* in the moment.

Self-Compassion and Interpersonal Skills

Self-compassionate people have been shown to be more effective in interpersonal relationships. People who were self-compassionate in one study were seen to be less judgmental, more accepting, and more connected with their partner than people who lacked self-compassion. Additionally, people with more self-compassion were more open to allowing their partner's autonomy and were encouraging of their partner's making their own decisions. It should be noted that self-compassion differs from self-esteem:

> Self-compassion fosters feeling of mutuality in relationships so that the needs of self and other are balanced and integrated. Self-esteem, on the other hand, is more ego-focused. (Neff, 2011, p. 221)

Self-Compassion, Self-Esteem, and Cultural Competence

In general, positive self-esteem implies an emphasis on positively *evaluating* some aspect(s) of ourselves. Many times we make this assessment through collecting opinions from others concerning a particular attribute. People with high self-esteem may have more confidence regarding relationships; however, they are not any more liked than people with average or lower self-esteem (Neff, 2011). Within a mindfulness perspective, we are sometimes cautioned against merely adopting "positive thinking" or affirmations regarding a personal characteristic or our overall worth. As mentioned earlier, Linehan (2005) asserts that this kind of approach is "dangerous" because it inevitably reinforces the activity of judging or thought replacement. We may judge ourselves as ugly, then look in the mirror and decide that we need to adjust this thinking and find a way to reduce our weight. Even if weight reduction is successful and is met with positive comments that on a self-esteem scale shows raised self-esteem, internal negative whispering may still be present. Any perceived sign in the external environment that appears to suggest negativity is viewed as a threat and may be met with hostility or despair because the self-esteem is still oriented to and rests on the fragile foundation of self- and other judgment.

Although DBT-WR clinicians should be cautious about both crafting interventions to "raise self-esteem" and providing positive affirmations, we should consider the dearth of positivity that some of our clients receive. As a result, we may consider balancing strengths-oriented language and praise with an awareness of the limitations of each. Carole Cartwright (personal interview, December 14, 2012) has a compelling perspective on this matter. Through leading DBT-informed practice groups for a crisis residential program, Ms. Cartwright has realized that her client base receives so much negativity about how and who they are—for example, mentally ill, drug addicted, poor, a person of color, crazy, a woman, a criminal, and homeless—that there is a need to "balance out" all the negativity. Her commitment as a therapist is to offer a loving presence and positive, affirming language because this kind of involvement is uplifting and so deeply appreciated by her clients. In addition to the general negativity that her clients have often internalized, so many clients have been abused, traumatized, abandoned, and betrayed. Joan Halifax (2008) describes modern-day society as "relationally depleted." People marginalized on the edges of our already depleted society and suffering with mental illness may particularly struggle from not feeling appreciated and valued.

The neutral language encouraged in DBT "to be mindful of self-judgments so as to see the thoughts as they are" does not address many of Ms. Cartwright's clients' needs to the degree that her active, direct, complimenting style does. Her method of active encouragement and practitioner emotional investment is designed to uplift the spirit and to demonstrate to her clients that someone is emotionally invested in their lives and in their corner.

Ms. Cartwright's affinity with her clients is impressive. As an African American woman who has a long history working with poor, dramatically underserved, and severely traumatized populations, her cultural slant on moving beyond the quietude that straight mindfulness practice sometimes involves is commendable and worthy of attention. When she shows her clients love, lets them know they are valued, tells them about the wonderful things she sees them do, and encourages them to see themselves as wonderful human beings, she asserts that they begin to manifest a twinkle in their eyes and a desire to do work. This *promising practice* may be more culturally consonant in various community settings where DBT-WR is applied.

Mindfulness of the Moment

Mindfulness practice is at the core of emotion regulation. As mentioned in Chapter 1, mindfulness helps us see our thoughts clearly so that they can have less power over us. Rather than be in the grip of troublesome thoughts, we have the opportunity to connect with our breath and get some space. As a result, we are less likely to perseverate or fuse with particular thoughts and *act out* with anger or *act in* with despair and self-harm. The multiple authors of a book on mindfulness and depression appreciate Jon Kabat-Zinn's simple definition of mindfulness: "Mindfulness means paying attention in a particular way on purpose, in the present moment, and non-judgmentally" (Segal, Williams, & Teasdale, 2002, p. 40).

In an attempt to more completely operationalize mindfulness as a psychological tool, Bishop et al. (2004) describe mindfulness as involving two components: (a) the self-regulation of attention; and (b) an orientation to present moment experience "characterized by curiosity, openness, and acceptance" (p. 232). Self-regulation of attention creates possibilities for observing thoughts and emotions and becoming acutely alert to here-and-now experience. Curiosity and acceptance create an environment of wonder and nonjudgment as well as the psychological predisposition to allow experience to unfold rather than to "push away" thoughts or emotions (Bishop et al., 2004).

In terms of our emotional process, we observe an agitated state and see, for example, anger arising. We learn from mindfulness exercises that our breath can ground us, and that the emotion of anger is not permanent and not as solid as we may imagine. We accept anger as an emotion and *make a decision about how to respond*. The capacity to see clearly and to skillfully choose a response enhances emotional regulation and utilizes the prefrontal cortex region of the brain, the part of the brain that helps us stay calm and effective. Demonstrating the brain regions to clients through an actual model or through an illustration (see Lesson 1 in Chapter 6) builds client enthusiasm and intention to engage in this work. Clients have been surprisingly empowered with the notion of neuroplasticity—that they can affect parts of the brain to become more or less active, inevitably leading to less reactivity and greater well-being.

Mindful acceptance of the immediate bodily sensations that arise in response to criticism, for example, helps us *stay* with our process and quiet the reactive internal voice that wants to immediately *do something* about the situation. Many times that "doing" reflex relates to a fight–flight–freeze response that is triggered by a rush of cortisol. Accepting the process may involve being aware of the inclination to react or aware of how the temperature of emotional life is beginning to heat up and set fire to emotional equilibrium. Accepting involves facing and being with this process. Staying with this process, making space for this process even in the face of some discomfort, is also part of acceptance. This quality of acceptance of thoughts and emotions is more likely if I am mindful of what the thoughts and emotions are; I am more mindful and can see the thoughts and feelings more clearly if I am accepting of their presence. The mutually reinforcing relationship between mindfulness and acceptance is experienced in a short mindfulness exercise.

Mindfulness Exercise

The mindfulness exercise instruction is to center our focus on an object, most often the breath. An object, like the breath, provides an opportunity to practice gathering our attention and developing facility for making contact with the present moment rather than "spacing out." The breath is an excellent object choice because it is always available to us and our attention to this embodied activity—breathing—helps quiet the mind, drop the ongoing narrative of our lives, and be in the present moment— where life is being lived. Rich opportunities for acceptance come largely, however, during the moments when attention leaves the connection with the breath. In those moments, there may or may not be mindfulness regarding the path that the mind is taking. When there is mindful recognition of ideas or feelings arising beyond the mindful attention to the breath, the job is to accept that this is where the mind is at this moment, and gently return to the breath. Acceptance is coming face-to-face with the reality of where your attention is. It is not about judging yourself for not doing a good job or, for that matter, judging yourself for doing a good job.

There are some people who will struggle with the traditional mindfulness activity of sitting while consistently bringing attention to the breath. The general rule is to have people notice their frustration with the activity and to accept their frustration. Thoughts about personal failure may arise as well as criticisms of mindfulness itself or of the clinician leading the exercise. Seeing these emotions and thoughts for what they are—thoughts and emotions that the clients do not need to attach to—can be part of the experience. In addition, you, as the practitioner, can normalize the degree to which people will bring their evaluative mind into this activity. It is positive for the client's "ratings" to be seen for what they are and to be dropped or released. This mindfulness instruction is a departure from the familiar cognitive approach for dealing with negative self-judgments, which is to replace our thoughts about being poor at something with thoughts about how good we are or how admirable we are for trying.

The final word on mindfulness practice is offered by Zen Master Dogen, who said that there is no such thing as good or bad meditation. This kind of encouragement—to let practice be as it is as well as to let the evaluative mind run its course—serves as a powerful metaphor for living life with greater emotional regulation and serenity. Imperfections, frustrations, judgments, self-judgments, bumps along the way, thoughts of "I got it this time; I am really good at this!" pass through while engaged in a mindfulness exercise. The thoughts, emotions, or experiences begin to be seen as insubstantial and transient and not to be taken so seriously. *We learn to radically accept whatever moves through the field and learn that this very acceptance reduces the charge of any particular thought or emotion.*

For people with thought disorders, settling and quieting the mind with a singular focus on breath may open the field for an intense awareness of auditory or visual hallucinations. The general rule of encouraging someone to grapple with some unpleasantness may not hold here. Some people with schizophrenia benefit greatly from some form of mindfulness, that is, developing capacity to see hallucinations as hallucinations that do not have to be believed; however, people who indicate that mindfulness work is too intense and wish to opt out should be respected for their self-assessment and allowed to do so. People may choose from a list of possibilities, including mindful walking (coordinating taking one step with an inhalation and one step with an exhalation), mindful drawing (focusing on the paper while maintaining some focus on breath for grounding), or mindfully chanting or repeating a phrase (can be silent chanting).

If you are leading a group with one or more members who struggle with traditional sitting meditation, then the group as a whole can receive exposure to various methods so as to minimize stigma for the person (or persons) who choose another mindfulness activity.

Overall, mindfulness work is about enhancing acceptance of self, other, one's emotional life, one's cognitive life, one's spiritual life, and the universe as it unfolds. The spirit of this work should mirror this stance of generosity and acceptance.

I am paraphrasing Zen teacher Edward Brown who has said while leading a meditation exercise, "I will ring the bell three times at the beginning and I will ring the bell two times at the end; whatever happens in between is called meditation." This statement urges us to drop ideas of performance, evaluation, comparison, and outcome regarding the endeavor of being with things as they are. We see where attention goes, we gently bring it back to the breath, and we accept the process that unfolds—even if the process includes nonaccepting thoughts, related irritations, daydreams, and periods of peace.

Mindfulness reduces the power of the judgmental mind. Even when this mind arises, there is an opportunity to accept that judgments have arisen and this process sets the ground for letting the judgments go. The word choice of *judgmental mind* and *judgments have arisen* is deliberately passive. Spend one minute with the intention of keeping your attention on the breath, and you will soon notice that your attention does not stay there. What becomes apparent during mindfulness exercises is that there is *not* an ego-like entity that has complete control over the mind's activity. Thoughts constantly come and go; what we learn through accepting their arrival and departure is not to become attached to the thoughts and not to become identified with the thoughts.

Judgments are one kind of thought. A mindful approach to a judgment is seeing it for what it is: a thought that can be let go and that does not need to be believed. As the focus returns to the breath and the lack of solidity or essence of a judgment becomes apparent, the judgment loses its grip on us. The same process occurs for self-judgments.

The terms to help describe acceptance—*being with, making space for, staying with*—as well as others are not easily comprehended with the rational mind. It is actual experience and practice with the concepts that teach us what they mean. Some clients may gravitate to one term or another to represent an experience, others will use terms of their own creation or refer to a situation or incident to symbolically capture an idea or concept. Some people prefer metaphors to make language such as *acceptance* feel real and meaningful; while the abstract quality of metaphors may be bothersome to others. Of course, one of the benefits of DBT-WR groups is that clients have the chance to witness how others are grappling with mindfulness and other DBT-WR ideas.

Meaning and Understanding of Mindfulness

Striking is the idiosyncratic way that people in DBT-WR groups articulated what mindfulness was and what it meant to them. Although their Kentucky Inventory of Mindfulness scores indicated significant changes in mindfulness, particularly on the dimension "acceptance without judgment" ($p < .001$) (Richards & Sehr, 2011), research respondents presented diverse statements explaining what mindfulness meant to them. Subjects who spoke of how mindfulness helped them deal with anger mentioned how important it was to be aware of emotions. For example:

> You don't have to blurt them out. Just go with the flow. That's how I took it. Be well mannered and you'll get on in life. Being aware of other people's feelings and how I say things. . . . We saw my boyfriend's son at the laundromat. He (my boyfriend) is really shy and won't say anything. I went up to his son and said hello and asked him where he worked. He said "somewhere" and then walked off. And I didn't come back with anything mean, which was different but good. I said, "all right," and then moved on. (Richards & Sehr, 2011, Subject 7, p. 59)

Another individual emphasized how important it was to link mindfulness to the experience in the body:

> Feeling the tension in the body (was important). Pay attention to the body, to the breathing. Be more aware. Know where it is so I can redirect it. So I can know what to do with it. If I don't know where it is, I don't know how to deal with it. (Richards & Sehr, 2011, Subject 16, p. 59)

One person talked about how mindfulness contributes to emotion regulation through *thoughtfulness*, which included for him/her a connection to the environment:

> I associate mindfulness with thoughtfulness. Like, when someone is speaking remember some rules like, "don't speak out of turn." You're mindful to be courteous to people. You are mindful to use your mind (laughs). To think about what you are going to say so that you can block some stuff out. You're mindful of the environment you might be in. So in that case mindfulness goes along

with awareness and thoughtfulness. Usually the mind in combination (with awareness and thoughtfulness). (Richards & Sehr, 2011, Subject 19, p. 60)

Finally, two people talked about how mindfulness enhanced their capacity for self-observation as it related to their specific mental health challenges:

Sometimes, because I'm bipolar, I have to be careful when I feel my mood swings coming on. Now, I can feel the immediate shifts in my mood, recognize and notice it without having to react to it (Richards & Sehr, 2011, Subject 2, p. 62).

Another subject who struggled with anxiety, depression, and substance abuse reported:

It (mindfulness) had a lot of meaning. It's like you're inside yourself and you could actually take time to focus on what you are feeling. You just focus on your breathing and you let go of stuff. It's so relaxing. It really is. It motivates you to want to get a second wind and keep going, and that helps you. (Richards & Sehr, 2011, Subject 3, p. 62).

Mindfulness as an Alternative Pathway

If I practice mindfulness and a coworker criticizes my work, I may notice thoughts arising regarding the legitimacy of the criticism, then thoughts directed at gaining perspective on the situation. "I am doing well at work . . . I am not sure where she is coming from . . . maybe over time we can work out whatever is coming between us." I may notice that I am feeling resentful that she brought this up, and then I uncover that the anger is a secondary emotion; the primary emotion (the emotion that is at the true core) is hurt. I notice that I am feeling less trusting, and that I have a thought that it may be helpful to get some space from her, at least for a while.

Without applying mindfulness, I may reactively experience anger, embarrassment, desire for revenge, and worry as a result of my coworker's criticism. I can start ruminating about "how dare she" accuse me of not being a good worker, when she herself is so . . . "I thought she was a friend I could count on . . . what an insensitive jerk she is." My anger could build as I think about the favors I have done for her, and about how ungrateful she is by comparison; then I could start worrying about whether she has revealed these so-called shortcomings to my boss and other coworkers. In the midst of anger, worry, hurt that I am not conscious of because I am too angry, and thoughts about being betrayed, I can start to feel despair. This event—my coworker's criticism—has taken over my life in this time period. I am in this dark hole, and there is nothing to do other than to take my shovel and dig it deeper. "Tonight I am going to go home and get loaded," I tell myself. The very contemplation of this behavior serves to bring relief in a manner, and is one of the few that I have at my disposal. Mindfulness is an effective tool to remediate the effects of the malfunctioning thermostat. With adequate mindfulness practice, the thermostat—the regulator of emotional life—reliably functions in order to steady the ship, address the choppy waters of life, and enhance emotional equilibrium.

Distress Tolerance

Distress tolerance is similar to the discussion of response modulation above. Linehan (1993) separates distress tolerance from emotion regulation in DBT to account for the presence of intense pain that may create risks to safety. In distress tolerance, the client learns to accept one's self, the situation, and his or her own pain as it arises. As we accept pain, we see it clearly and realize we do not have to add a story to it or magnify it with worry. (As the coworker story unfolded in the preceding example, we can see how I may become progressively distressed.) If this case had been true and I had been experiencing significant emotion regulation challenges, I would pursue one of the crisis survival strategies that Linehan (1993) emphasized: acceptance, distracting, self-soothing, and improving the moment.

Responding to Emotions in the Moment

There are various ways to regulate one's emotions (see Gross & John, 2003; Gross & Thompson, 2007). *Situation selection* refers to choosing environments or scenarios that are more likely to produce positive emotions. Being with someone who sometimes directs hurtful comments toward you may offer the benefit of feeling less lonely, but often leaves you feeling small, insecure, and ashamed. Maybe choosing another friend or activity would be preferable in the name of emotion regulation and taking care of yourself.

The next three strategies are to be implemented once a person is in the middle of a situation that is unfolding. *Situation modification* involves making conscious changes to a given situation before intense emotions arise. As I contemplate writing, for example, I notice my own process of rumination and creeping despair entering my emotional field. I modify my situation of being at home alone, beginning to perseverate, and procrastinating through watching television, and I modify the situation. I decide to make tea, open the laptop, and start working. In this case, I am generating movement toward working and am initiating effort in the service of not only making progress and fulfilling a responsibility, but also in the service of personal emotional regulation. Recent anecdotes with university and high school students who suffer from stress regarding work completion show promise for a mindful approach to procrastination. Instead of battling with what they "should do" with their time, feeling shame during the time they are not working, feeling anxious as a deadline approaches, and seeming to require a massive infusion of stress in order to mobilize themselves to move beyond the cycle of resentment and shame, students are asked whether they wish to approach assignment timelines from the perspective of emotion regulation strategies vis-à-vis their stress level and sense of wellness.

A mindful approach to situation modification means that students learn to notice and accept times that they have thoughts or feelings regarding work completion. Once doing so, they learn to enjoy their non-homework time and let go of the lingering thoughts regarding how they "should be" doing something else. Involvement with work completion proceeds as a skillful response for taking care of one's self, and thus involves **self-compassion**. This approach to working with deadlines represents an example of how situation modification may be applied.

The final two strategies that help with emotion regulation while situations are unfolding are *attentional deployment* and *cognitive change*. Attentional deployment refers to how we direct our attention in order to affect our emotions. In one extensive experiment of infant boys and girls, girls seemed to have greater facility for attentional deployment when infants were faced with their mother's sudden withdrawal of eye contact and active verbal communication (Thompson, 2006). Representative video evidence depicted girls being more able to shift their attention to their surroundings and points within the room, while infant boys had less facility to refocus attention. As a result of this differential, boys manifested less ability to self-soothe. In terms of older adults, you may assist your own emotion regulation if you did not focus attention on distressing people or situations you could not control such as worries about a family member's health.

Cognitive change is another strategy that helps regulate our emotions during situations. We gain perspective of a situation and issue a statement to ourselves to help define or explain a situation in order to reduce distress. If a person is grouchy with us, we may tell ourselves that the person actually still feels good about us and that he or she is just having a bad day. We rationally gather information and realize that we are not in danger of being abandoned, being fired, or being disliked. We are not to blame for what is happening. Such a cognitive strategy may enhance our sense of safety and reduce our sense of vulnerability.

Response modulation is unique from the four strategies discussed above because response modulation comes into play *after* an emotion-generating response has already developed. The modulation is focused on regulating the physiological response or behavioral response that has unfolded and often involves suppression of emotionally charged behavior. It is believed that the four "antecedent-focused" emotion regulation strategies mentioned above are associated with overall well-being more than response modulation (Schutte, Manes, & Malouff, 2009).

Mindfulness may affect one's capacity to select situations, to prevent reactive responses in the midst of situations, or to modulate emotional responses as they arise. Mindful observation involving curiosity and openness is dispassionate. It is thought that

> [t]his dispassionate state of self observation . . . introduce(s) a "space" between one's perception and response. Thus mindfulness is thought to enable one to respond to situations more reflectively (as opposed to reflexively) [parentheses in original quote]. (Bishop et al., 2004, p. 232)

In the freedom of this space, clients can make choices about how to respond. Not so hijacked by emotion, or victimized by environmental cues that trigger habitual, patterned behavior, a person may notice her or his internal process unfold and sense that she or he is empowered to take care of one's self. This

Responding	Reacting
Fueled by intention to be in Wise Mind	Limited intention regarding Wise Mind
Acknowledging of thoughts and emotions that arise	Not mindful of emotional states
Sorting out how thoughts lead to emotions and emotions lead to thoughts	Stirred by emotions. Build cognitive structures that fuel emotions further
Maintaining intention to care for self and others	Not having conscious intention or losing sight of the intention to care for self and others
Stay with experience and accept experience as it is	Deny experience, space out, or seek immediate solution
Choose skillful response based upon self-care, commitment for growth, and values	Reactivity governed by fight-freeze-flight or habitual patterns
Pre-frontal cortex based	Amygdala based
May have spiritual context; e.g., "this is part of my awakening, part of my path"	"Get this out of my life!"
Movement toward being with and opening to	Movement to conflict/avoidance dichotomy
Emotion regulation, seeking support	Feeling ashamed, guilty, angry, and isolating
Mindful distraction	Denial
Breath-based and patient	Reactivity-based and hurried, impulsive
Rests on foundation of self-compassion	Rests on foundation of fear and habit

Figure 2.2   Responding vs. Reacting

ability to respond lends itself to the notion that the client has "response-ability" or responsibility for how the unfolding of emotions leads to behavioral responses. The contrast between responding and reacting is depicted in Figure 2.2.

Anecdotally, I have seen the promise for reducing reactivity and, particularly, emotionally reactivity-inspired behavior as a result of this approach. For years my supervisees and I have worked with clients struggling with posttraumatic stress disorder (PTSD) and have had unproductive, after-the-fact reflections with these clients concerning their various behaviors.

A simplistic version of a common client–clinician conversation follows:

Practitioner: So you did X last night, how helpful was doing X for you?

Client: I really shouldn't have done that. It made things worse and now I am in more trouble than before.

Practitioner: So what do you take away from all this?

Client: I really don't want to act this way again. I'm not sure why I get so angry, but next time I do, I will make sure not to do such dumb stuff.

Practitioner: Okay. It's good that you can learn from this and that you are committed to be less impulsive. It's good that you can see that, first, you were upset and then you did X. Maybe next time you are upset you can call a friend or something so you won't get into trouble. You seem committed to your recovery.

Client: Thank you.

Whether working with youth or adults, it seems that conversations like these frequently have limited effect. There may even be sincere client intentions to more skillfully respond to environmental situations and arising emotions; however, without the kind of emotion regulation training that is present in DBT-WR, the foundation of client skills is not available to call upon in the moment when a situation sparks a reactive sequence.

Responding With Letting Go

Letting go may become a mantra for living a life in peace and in accord with the way things are. Ultimately, we become emotionally and spiritually mature when we realize that we do not have control over the ways people act, the fact that we will age, and the reality that people will come and go in our lives. To some extent, although we are training in emotion regulation, we cannot even fully control the arising of emotional states. Letting go is a practice that we may adopt as a general approach to life as well as a **respond to the moment** skill to regulate our emotions.

> [L]etting go liberates us from (a) our difficult past experiences and seemingly unmanageable lives; (b) our stuck and sometimes distorted (or in the 12-step tradition— "stinking") thinking involving personal judgment and shame; (c) rigid (or reactive) emotional states like despair, resentment, or anger; and (d) patterns of behavior or relationships that are not healthy or fulfilling. (Bein, 2008, p. 59)

Some people are assisted with the cognitive and spiritual lessons embedded in the serenity prayer, the ultimate reminder for letting go:

> God, grant me the serenity
> To accept the things I cannot change;
> The courage to change the things I can;
> And the wisdom to know the difference.

The medicine for accepting what cannot be changed is letting go. Let go of the idea that your will, your desire to have things be different, your ideas about unfairness, your plans, your temper tantrums and frustrations, and your schemes will be enough to make the world fit your image of the way it should be or the way you want it to be.

On some level there is a subtle letting go as we mindfully meet the moment with radical acceptance. We radically accept that the entire history of the universe has led up to this very moment; thus, to one degree or another, this moment's manifested nature has been caused. Some may say this moment was "meant to be" either—depending on spiritual orientation— because causes and conditions have evolved in such a manner that the moment logically manifested (thinking in accord with Eastern thought/Karma or humanism) or that it was meant to be because God or Allah has divined it to be so. Some people reject the language of "meant to be," and may even find it alienating. On the most pragmatic and inclusive level, we radically accept that what has happened, has happened. There is no way to re-create the past and change the fact that you are reading this sentence right now!

Radical acceptance means radical acceptance of everything. Rewriting the Serenity Prayer in this spirit would mean that we would wish to be granted the serenity to *accept it all*— whether we can change it or not. Accept that we either can or cannot change some things. And accept that we may sometimes have the wisdom to know what we may change and other times we may be "wisdom-challenged" and discern incorrectly whether change is possible.

We radically accept emotions, thoughts, and situations, as well as how difficult it is to radically accept. Again, radical acceptance is coming face to face with the truth; it does not imply approval or passivity in the face of oppression. The radically accepting person says, "Yes, this is happening," and thus is *more likely* to effectively respond than the person who is in denial or is deluded about what is taking place. In radical acceptance we let go of the fight against reality. We see clearly and then do not get on the reactivity train taking us on a wild ride filled with stories, righteousness, anger, and diminished clarity regarding our potential to make a difference.

With radical acceptance we let go of the superfluous, and we open, with curiosity, to the reality of life. We approach ourselves and others with an open hand rather than a clenched fist, and we incline toward kindness and understanding. We let go over and over again of the stories and narratives that are often so present that we mistake their buzzing chatter for our actual lives.

Cultural Interface With Radical Acceptance

Some people inevitably equate radical acceptance with passivity. It may be easy to recite an example showing how radical acceptance means directly facing a situation, such as in the case where one partner is experiencing physical abuse from another. Within this example, the argument is made that the person who radically accepts this abuse as well as the pain experienced—in other words, the person who does not deny or bargain about the dynamics and consequences of the abuse—is the person who will be prepared to be most responsive. *Docility or approval is not implied with radical acceptance.* Despite this explanation, some people who have suffered historical oppression do not appreciate the radical acceptance terminology. I have had African Americans tell me that no matter what I say about radical acceptance, they will not, for example, "accept" slavery. Larry Yang, LCSW, core teacher at a multicultural, inner-city meditation center, as well, has discussed with me the emotional charge that acceptance language has for some attendees, particularly people of color.

DBT-WR that is culturally competent should furnish access points available to all. For this reason, "radically facing reality," "showing up for what is," and "radical non-reactivity" are offered as alternatives that: (a) seems less objectionable, (b) validate and demonstrate empathy regarding personal experiences and orientations that are different, and (c) model radical acceptance (or facing reality) of people's often marginalized world views.

Responding With Soothing

At times our emotional life is challenging for us even, sometimes, to the degree that our overall well-being is threatened. We are mindful of the level of distress present in our lives and how attempts at letting go may not be effective. We realize that we need to care for ourselves, sometimes in the way that a caring and healthy parent would care for a sick child. It is important to identify activities or situations that can fulfill this role either as a preventative, resilience-building measure or as a coping tool to draw upon in the midst of distress.

Some have utilized various soothing strategies that have served as a temporary fix, but, in the long run, may have created additional suffering. We may have attempted to soothe ourselves with drugs, or indulged in some form of self-harm like cutting to relieve pain, and found that though these strategies served a function, they had various pitfalls and often times made our overall situation worse.

Identifying self-soothing strategies is important because in the midst of experiencing difficulties, utilizing this list may help us stay safe. Additionally, strategies that can create self-harm, like drug use, may be compelling in times of difficulty. In fact, painful emotions can be a trigger to use or to engage in a cycle of further rumination and contemplation of self-harm or suicide. Self-soothing strategies such as taking a bath, going on Facebook, or drinking tea may serve to reduce distress and enhance moment-to-moment safety for some clients. In some instances it may be important to incorporate harm reduction principles to create the self-soothing list. Items, such as holding an ice cube (rather than cutting), or eating one dessert (instead of binging), are illustrations.

Thought defusion may be employed as a soothing strategy (Luoma, Hayes, & Walter, 2007). This process involves building capacity to mindfully see a thought and to reduce the thought's centrality and influence on our lives. For example, we may hold a thought that has a self-critical charge for us. Our task is to notice it as a thought rather than the truth; it is mental activity, nothing more. The next instruction is to imagine a scenario where the thought could be transported away—a leaf moving downstream, a cloud floating away— then develop an image of the object carrying away the thought.

Responding With Engaging in Positive Action

Engaging in positive action not only helps in coping with troubling emotions, it serves as a protective factor that prevents distress from arising. While being *mindful* of boredom or restlessness—emotional states that may be precursors to more intense emotional states like despair or agitation—one may develop an intention to engage in something positive in order to ward off troublesome emotions. In general, it is important to not only increase positive experiences but to be mindful of these experiences (Marra, 2004). The mind that is engaged in an increased number of events that involve emotions related to *love, joy, mastery,* and *calmness* is less vulnerable to experiencing distressing emotions and more adept at dealing with troublesome emotions when they do arise.

Additionally, although it is not encouraged to create a story regarding "how good the day was," we inevitably do this. A day involving mindfully engaged positive action stacks up better, in review, than a day in which we operated predominantly on automatic pilot. In other words, if at the end of the day we find ourselves agitated and dealing with arising distressing emotions, it may be helpful to include in the mental review how we had a conversation with a friend and rode our bike, rather than have the review be "I sat at home and watched TV."

The deliberate listing of positive actions assists in consistently executing them. Again, the instruction is to be mindfully present while undertaking various elements on the list. The list may include subtle and easy-to-access elements of life. For *love,* spending time with a person, sharing experiences, having good communication, and feeling some connection—whether with nature, a pet, or spirituality—are possibilities. For *joy,* being accepted, having pleasurable sensations, being involved in a rewarding activity are points of orientation. *Mastery* involves a sense of "I can do this," or "I am okay," or "I am part of things." These kinds of experiences can come from being involved in a 12-step community, engaging in art, assisting someone, taking a class, or doing something positive at work. Developing calmness involves cultivating a sense of being comfortable with who you are and with your body. Paying attention to breath, living your commitment to take care of yourself, taking a yoga or mindfulness-based stress reduction (MBSR) class, and maintaining your intention to implement the DBT-WR exercises contribute to the cultivation of calmness.

Responding With Opposite Action

Opposite action is a cognitive-behavioral intervention that breaks destructive emotion–response sequences that the client may be inclined to engage in (Linehan, 1993). The responses that flow from emotions may be ineffective or unskillful for two reasons. First, the response or behavior is the final link in the *reactive* chain of thought–emotion–behavior. As an example, if someone does not text me back right away, I think about how he does not really care about me; I feel insecure, abandoned, and enraged; I text him an inflammatory message about what a jerk he is.

Second, emotions may lead to unskillful behavior because there are situational cues, which include the emotional environment, that bring on habitual or patterned behavior. In the face of boredom, I may routinely leave the house and look for people to drink with. Or when my partner asks me to do the dishes, I think that the request is unfair and is part of my partner's nagging and harassing me, so I get angry and yell at her to go do them herself.

Opposite action is a pithy instruction that has powerful consequences when acted upon. Rather than the clinician's implicitly criticizing the client for acting inappropriately, opposite action directs the client to consider another approach— opposite of the usual—for responding to the moment. Mindfulness is needed in order to notice arising emotion and to provide a space for the client to consider a behavioral alternative that stretches the person's behavioral repertoire. Taking action in this new, opposite from usual direction creates outcomes that move the person toward greater wellness.

At times (as shown in Lesson 6, Chapter 6), the decision to engage in opposite action may spark someone to take to take a healthy risk. In the midst of anxiety, for example, one may normally decide to stay away from people and not reach out. Someone can notice this process unfold: I feel anxious; I want to stay away from people so the anxiety will not get worse. The underlying message embedded in opposite action is that our reactive and familiar responses actually make us suffer more. We stay away because we are afraid, so we become more afraid of social situations and deprive ourselves of potential support. Or we yell when we are frustrated and stressed, and we create more frustration and stress through yelling.

Opposite action practice does not only create more skillful behavioral possibilities, it also enhances our Wise Mind through cultivating a positive feedback loop of noticing and accepting thoughts and emotions, calming reactivity and habitual response patterns, and choosing wellness-oriented behavior.

Cognitive Lessons and Secondary Emotions

There are principles about emotions that are important to explore and that normalize people's experience with emotions. These principles also assist the client to adopt a radically accepting, nonjudgmental stance to emotional experience. There are certain myths about emotions that are widely held. These myths may be reinforced as truths in environments that are particularly invalidating or that in one way or another communicate that there is little room for the expression of one's internal life. Such myths are that (a) there is a right way to feel in every situation; (b) letting people know how I feel is weakness; (c) all painful emotions are the result of a bad attitude; and (d) if others do not approve of my feelings, I should not feel the way I do (Linehan, 1993).

One's experience of trauma (as we will discuss in Chapter 4) often involve b, c, and d. Painful emotions are invalidated or denied. There is something wrong with me for having them. In the long run, it would be better to stuff my feelings and keep my mouth shut.

Other elements for consideration help one embrace emotions and see their value rather than to view emotions as "the enemy." Linehan (1993) directs clients to understand that emotions help to communicate and develop intimacy with others. They are part of our internal life and we may be able to make our needs known as we tune into them. Emotions prepare us for action, for example, our compassion to reach out to others or enthusiasm to achieve a goal. Finally, we are hard-wired to experience emotions. Noticing them and accepting them is *self-validating*. They may be giving us vital information—in the form of signals or alarms—that will keep us safe.

The discussion of primary and secondary emotions also helps clients develop a wider understanding of their emotional life. Through this cognitive pathway, clients may be able to tap into, reveal, and deal with previously obscured emotions. "Secondary emotions are complicated, non-adaptive patterns of emotions *about* emotions" (Spradlin, 2002, p. 27). Secondary emotion patterns may have emerged because it has felt safer, in terms of family or wider social context, to experience and express these emotions rather than emotions that are primary ones. Often, we take action based on a felt sense of our secondary emotions and create more difficulty and suffering.

A common secondary emotion is anger. Anger provides cover for the primary emotion (i.e., the authentic emotion) of sadness or hurt. In many families, one became too vulnerable if she or he said, "I am hurt (or sad) by what happened." The feeling morphed into anger about a perceived or experienced transgression. In a family situation where members did not take responsibility for how they may have contributed to someone's being hurt, or who laughed at someone's vulnerability, it made sense to become angry. Although Spradlin (2002) uses the term *nonadaptive* to characterize secondary emotions, these kinds of emotions probably arose because at one time they were, in fact, adaptive. Secondary emotions may also relate to socially prescribed ways of behaving along gender lines. It may be that for men, expressing anger is more permissible than sadness or fear, while for women, expressing the secondary emotion of sadness or despair may be more socially acceptable than anger.

The revelation of primary and secondary emotions allows clients in DBT-WR to gain glimpses of their more complex emotional selves. Instead of, for the sake of the stereotype, a man's lashing out against a person who has wronged him, he may have the chance to venture into the softer emotional world of feeling helpless or sad. Sometimes in this emotional space, acknowledgment, validation, and increased confidence to hold personal sadness allows one to back off from the reactive behavioral response that flows from and perpetuates anger. (It is important to emphasize that this characterization is a gender stereotype. Many women have the same propensity to emphasize anger, particularly, in my experience, women suffering from PTSD.)

The following are possibilities where secondary emotions make their appearance and obscure primary emotions:

Despair about sadness
Anger about sadness or hurt
Shame for being embarrassed
Self-loathing for being sad
Guilt about being contented
Anxiety about joy ending/grief
Anger about fear
Sadness about fear

The identification and exploration of secondary emotions contributes to enhanced emotional regulation because the client is able to mindfully accept and see clearly her or his previously obscured emotional life. Responding to this deeper, more profound, picture yields responses that are more about self-care and skillfulness and less about habit and reaction.

Expanding the Moment: Resilience Building and the Bigger Picture

Emotion regulation efforts may also be directed toward building individual resilience and personal protective factors. If clients are willing to engage with life (rather than embodying willfulness which opposes engagement), and their day is filled with satisfying activities, positive relationships, and the intention and follow-through to be self-compassionate and self-soothing, a sense of well-being and enhanced emotional life results. The steady presence of positive experiences as well as confidence that one can ride the waves of pleasure and pain reinforces that life is worth living. Many ride the waves of pleasure and pain through their capacity to touch "the bigger picture" at various points in their day. This connection helps people move beyond what is referred to as the "small mind," in other words, the mind that is frequently worried about what is going to happen to me and acts like my thoughts and emotions are the totality of existence. At times, it is difficult to regulate emotions when there is little spaciousness in the universe and no "place to go" other than one's perceptual and emotional experience of reality.

The Cultivation of Hope

Resilience building is in accord with a mental health recovery orientation that we will cover in greater detail later. For now, a few elements are discussed that are to be incorporated into the DBT-WR emotion-regulation model presented here. The first resilience-building element is hope. "Hope is the catalyst of the recovery process . . . (and) provides the essential message of a better future, that consumers can overcome the obstacles confronting them as they pursue psychological growth" (Walsh, 2013, p. 17). Not only is client or consumer hope important for recovery but we, as providers, are encouraged to help the client internalize it (Walsh, 2013). Although the discussion of hope is fundamental knowledge for helping professionals, there is no explicit mention of cultivating hope within DBT.

In general, DBT's emphasis on mindfulness and acceptance likely precludes including the cultivation of hope as an important skill. From the Eastern or Buddhist view that is part of DBT's foundation, hope is seen as emphasizing the act of waiting for (in fact, the Spanish word *esperar* means to hope or to *wait for*) something better to happen. This "waiting for" element seems to contrast with the DBT skill of noticing, accepting, and dealing with what actually arises in the present moment. Therefore, following this line of reasoning, placing emotional investment into a better future may imply a lack of intention for accepting things as they are. Additionally, a core DBT skill is to develop confidence and capacity to deal with situations, thoughts, and emotion states as they arise. We maintain awareness and involvement in the present moment with an accompanying sense that the way in which the future unfolds is very much out of control and has not yet arrived. Hope may be seen as attempting to bring the future into the present, consequently leading clients to adopt unhealthy attachments to particular future results.

I have implemented a relatively hope-free stance regarding the progression of my daughter's schizophrenia, for example. This stance has helped me stay present and connected with her regardless of how well she is doing or how much she is struggling. This disease as well as other life challenges have taught me to roll with whatever life puts in my begging bowl—to use a Zen metaphor—and to not get too attached as to whether the bowl contains an ample, well-prepared Thai meal or a few kibbles of dog food.

I still look to support my daughter's aspirations and to be there for her in any way that I can. I would like nothing more than to help her live a life worth living. Engaging in "non-hope" does not preclude me or my partner from researching medications that may be more efficacious or about social or educational opportunities that may contribute to Emily's happiness. Of course, I want the best for her, but not relying on hope has helped me feel confident of my capacity to deal with whatever unfolds and to not become emotionally reactive when the begging bowl yields just a few morsels of hard-to-digest food.

Despite my own engagement in nonhope and the degree to which a DBT program would not explicitly include hope, hope's importance is championed in the mental health recovery literature (Slade, 2009; Walsh, 2013).

> Hope . . . involves not only positive expectancies and specific goals of agency but also the flexibility to respond to obstacles by changing goals or methods. . . . A 5-week hope focused orientation group for people starting to use a community mental health center led to benefits in relation to well-being, functioning, coping, and symptomology, especially for clients with lower initial hope. (Slade, 2009, pp. 129–130)

When times are especially painful, emotions are raw, and anger, grief, and despair have taken over, making the tunnel appear completely dark, a glimmer of hope offers a reason to take one step forward. The energy required to try the next medication, and the next one, and the next one; to reach out to a family member or friend to say "please help"; to attend the next DBT-WR group or attempt a therapy exercise; to get out of bed the next day; to apply for financial or housing assistance with a government program deliberately designed to discourage the applicant; to walk to the store to buy cigarettes even though people may look at you funny; to enter a relationship even though many relationships before have produced pain;

to navigate through troublesome thoughts, feelings, and situations—that energy's source is hope.

Contemplating about hope in my daughter's life, I have an image of the sun pouring into the car as we took a familiar drive down the delta. As my daughter sang, her voice would rise above her sometimes grinding depression. She was experiencing frightening, unrelenting symptoms; she was not in a relationship; and she was not sure whether life was worth living, but her voice expressed a touch of joy and a sense of connection. She always thanked my partner and me deeply during those many drives. Those drives were a lifeline, something that gave shape to the day and hope that life had something to offer. Eventually, there was hope about going to school and attending community college, hope about being in a relationship, hope that some combination of medication would help, and hope about making a contribution. Hope sustained her as she persevered through various obstacles: an intense relationship fell apart, school was interrupted by hospitalization, medications needed to be changed because of either horrible side effects or lack of effectiveness, and psychiatrists needed to be changed for some of the same reasons.

Additionally, hope, singing, music, sunlight, and companionship served to regulate painful emotions and distress. I learned later that, at times, my daughter requested these drives when she was intensely struggling and had self-destructive fantasies. During these moments in the car, friends that she would see in the future and upcoming TV episodes were briefly discussed. During these drives, life was pretty okay. There was something to look forward to; maybe life would get better at some point; maybe life was worth living for another day.

Marsha Linehan's videos are filled with hopeful comments. "The good news is you can do it," she says (Linehan, 2005). I wasn't so good at mindfulness and I learned; you can learn, too. At the conclusion of her mindfulness video, she asks the question, "Do you want to be free?" What can be more motivating for engaging in mindfulness practice than the hopeful possibility that, first, I can do it despite my initial struggles, and, second, I can be free.

Emotion regulation, then, would seem to be facilitated through client hopefulness. Ultimately, a basketball player shoots the same shots thousands of times because that player believes that practicing the skill leads to improvement—so hope becomes the incentive for staying the course. Accepting and mindfully being in the present and the experience of hopefulness are dialectically related. They may appear to oppose each other, but as all dialectically related elements, they are actually two sides of the coin. We engage in mindfulness because we are hopeful of positive benefits; we are mindful and accepting of our hopefulness, and we are less subject to being thrown about and knocked off center by arising thoughts, feeling states, or situations. Paradoxically, then, our mindful practice and capacity for emotion regulation strengthens and is strengthened by hopefulness even though hope, itself, is embedded with the pitfall of orienting us toward the future.

Emotional dysregulation contributes to hopelessness. When our life experience is dominated by fluctuating, painful, and out-of-control emotions, then life seems to be a series of crises and ongoing misery. One wave after another hits us, and we barely make it up for air. Life becomes exhausting, and people around us may become exhausted being with us. The kind of serenity available to some seems elusive, so life does not seem to have a resting point; a place where a deep wisdom or connection to something greater than the small self brings peace.

Expanding the Moment and Spirituality

Many people rely on spirituality in order to experience well-being and live with serenity and hopefulness. Marsha Linehan herself has recently spoken about how, during dark times, a spiritual experience turned *her* life around and set her on a path that in essence meant there was "no going back." By this she meant not ever returning to a life where she felt unloved and where she was hopelessly lost (see New York Times Video, 2011).

Spirituality is a liberating force for many clients. Many lean on their religious and spiritual life to provide meaning, direction, hopefulness, serenity, and happiness (Canda, Nakashima, & Furman, 2004; Hodge, 2005). It makes sense to systematically incorporate spirituality into DBT because of its potential for healing and its contribution to moment-to-moment emotional regulation. There is greater likelihood for reactivity when a particular situation, thought, or mood state fills up one's world, and the person's experienced world fuses with these elements. A glimpse to the skies above, to a universal sense of beauty, a connection with grace, gratitude, or love, or to one's deepest purpose creates possibilities that life contains more than the stimulus–response, emotionally reactive universe of the amygdala. Such a view is embraced in the substance abuse world where recovery centers on a connection to "something greater than self" in order to move one beyond a world dominated by craving and small-minded action.

Let us address the various challenges to incorporating spiritual view squarely within a DBT framework. The first involves confusion about the difference between spirituality and religion. The second challenge includes the issue of people being turned off to religion and spirituality. Religious practices have, in fact, wounded some (see Bein, 2008), while others are generally alienated by these matters. Finally, because of the diversity of spiritual and religious experiences, values, and attitudes, inclusive and nonalienating language is important to offer different pathways for clients. This model's use of "expanding the moment" and "bigger picture" will be discussed.

Spirituality and Religion Defined

The term *spirituality* conjures up various thoughts and emotional reactions. Some will restrict the discussion of spirituality to the realm of one's experience with her or his higher power.

Exploring spirituality thus needs to incorporate questions regarding the ways in which one understands, makes contact with, and is guided through the higher power's presence. People speak about realizing that their higher power or God deeply loves them for who they are, and they may feel the benefits of serenity that come from believing that there is a reason that they are on the planet. At the very least, some part of this reason often includes doing work on God's or their higher power's behalf.

Alcoholics Anonymous (AA) to some degree acknowledged the challenges that members may have for relating to God. They prepared people on the second of the 12 steps to consider that a "power greater than ourselves could restore us to sanity" (Wilson & Smith, 1939). In the following step, they label that power as "God" but allow for some flexibility, with "God as we understood him." Although founded by Christian men, early AA visionaries extended the net to create some access for non-Christians. People who do not consider themselves particularly Christian or religious continue to struggle with 12-step programs. In the conventional AA language, "God" is explicitly mentioned four times through the 12 steps and the male pronoun or possessive "him" or "his" is also used four times (Wilson & Smith, 1939). Although not to be explored in detail here, the Lord's Prayer, which has Christian roots, is usually recited at the end of 12 step meetings and causes additional consternation among various attendees.

When 12-step attendees struggle with language and program orientation, members, sponsors, and treatment providers problem solve in order to develop personal interpretations that work in the 12-step environment. The term *higher power* is zeroed in on, and participants learn that there are many possibilities. People may think of the AA or Narcotics Anonymous (NA) fellowship as a higher power, while others incorporate the view that love, itself, is a higher power. "The universe's" patterns, creations, awe-inspiring essence, and unknown quality are higher power elements that people resonate with.

In addiction, the thinking goes, the substance or the addiction process has gained prominence in one's life. Surrendering to the reality of personal powerlessness in the face of an evolving "life (that) has become unmanageable" (Wilson & Smith, 1939) means that one has to be oriented toward making room for a force greater than self to enter and assist. The self, left to its own devices, has not been up to the task.

An evolving intention toward emotion regulation offers some interesting parallels and differences. On some level, we begin to make progress when we admit that emotion dysregulation has caused pain, and, up until this point, our own efforts and strategies to manage emotions—stay unaware, repress, act out, engage in self-harm, rely on secondary emotions such as anger and rage rather than feeling sad and vulnerable—are not serving us. We accept our reality and understand that receiving help can make a difference.

Within the skills of traditional DBT, prayer is listed as one among many distress tolerance strategies (Linehan, 1993); however, wide-ranging spirituality is not conceptualized as a protective factor for resilience or a sanctuary in the midst of arising dysregulation.

Spirituality as a Quest for Meaning and a Tool Against Stigma

Various conceptualizations of spirituality make the topic broadly approachable and inclusive (see Canda et al., 2004). Spirituality for some involves *a quest for meaning*. Why am I here . . . do I have a contribution to make? is a possible question within this vein. Some may have abandoned this quest because they have come to believe social or familial messages that they have so little to offer the world or that their presence on the planet has been a sorry mistake.

Societal stigma enhances the idea of inferiority for many clients who have been marginalized to one extent or another. Regarding those with mental illness, stigma contributes mightily to low feelings of self worth and diminished motivation to move forward with treatment (Davidson, Tondora, Lawless, O'Connell, & Rowe, 2009):

> What advocates within the mental health community have come to call "internalized stigma" presents a significant obstacle to recovery, undermining the self-confidence and self-esteem required for the person to take steps toward improving his or her life. The demoralization and despair that are associated with internalized stigma and feelings of inferiority also sap the person's sense of hope and initiative, adding further weight to the illness and its effects. (pp. 131–132)

Clients who struggle with mental illness deal with persistent familial, societal, and interpersonal rejection that interacts with the client's own emotional and mental instability. While the mutually reinforcing relationship between mental health challenges and rejecting, demeaning, or volatile social interactions continues, people attempt to cope through social isolation or through connecting with others over the use of substances. (Dual diagnosis demographics will be presented later.)

Strengthening the client view of personal worthlessness derived from social stigma as well as from challenging, conflictual, and sometimes violent relationships are the clients' own personally held beliefs about themselves. Clients may equate receiving assistance for their mental health disability and their not holding as job as indicative of their lower value. Their ethnic/racial background, sexual orientation, cognitive or behavioral issues, or the fact that they have been either mandated or pushed into receiving counseling are elements that may find their way into the mix of an internalized sense of inferiority.

The search for meaning and grappling with one's contribution to the world open avenues for healing, hope, and a fresh view. One lesson involves looking at the ways that the client's job is to be well, relate to others positively, and to inspire others as they progress along the path. Although making money is heavily valued in the society, we examine the degree to which self-honesty, the willingness to learn and apply mindfulness, and a commitment to respond to the world in a healthy manner dramatically contributes to society. I discuss with my clients the degree to which I, myself, am inspired watching people's honesty, heart, and sincere effort.

Some people may connect this search for meaning to—as one client said—"being the person that God wanted me to be." Others may discuss what being a loving, consistent, and caring family member means; some people want to contribute to the 12-step community; some want to create art; some feel that appreciating the world creates positive ripples; some want to live in peace moment-to-moment; some embrace the value and contribution of telling the truth; and some are making plans to go to school or get their GED, look for work, or act with greater integrity in the job they currently possess.

The practitioner's job, then, is to deconstruct society's usual methods for evaluating worth, and to genuinely and deeply appreciate the client's journey and the client's own emerging sense of value and contribution. This cognitive process sets the stage for and enhances an exploration into spiritual elements related to one's fundamental goodness and worthiness for living "a life worth living." As the client internalizes (a) the practitioner's appreciation of the client's courage; (b) the practitioner's unconditional support and caring as well as the *absence* of connecting affection and admiration with client role acquisition or performance; (c) the practitioner's manifested belief that the world is better off due to the existence of the person; and (d) the practitioner's radical acceptance (as opposed to denigration) of diverse client personal characteristics, the cognitive deconstruction of "contribution" and "worth" merges with a larger spiritual view (Bein, 2008).

In addition to the acceptance-related behaviors of the clinician, a willingness to explicitly explore client spirituality and embrace the client's own version of the bigger picture set the stage for developing a foundation of spiritual resources that can be accessed while implementing the strategy of *expand the moment*.

For clients suffering from PTSD and emotional distress symptoms that arise throughout the day (Briere & Scott, 2006), a wider view may assist coping. In one such case, I spoke with a man recently diagnosed with PTSD and mentioned that I *admired his courage* to persist in seeking the truth about his life and in ascertaining how to live a fulfilling life. "Thank you for saying that," he said. "Most of the time I think about how people are probably thinking about how lazy I am."

We can look at this exchange as a simple practitioner reframe, in other words, a cognitive intervention designed for the person to internalize a new message about himself. What the exchange entailed was a bigger picture view of this delightful, open-hearted person who also happens to struggle in life. In this moment, he was completely seen and acknowledged as precious and inspirational. Exchanges of smiles and deep thank-yous laid the groundwork for more exploration. What will you do with this one precious life? How do you contribute to others? Perhaps some of the following client suppositions or contemplations are invoked: "Maybe my life has some purpose"; "Maybe God or a higher power put me in this position/gave me these challenges so I can teach others"; "Maybe I am loved by the universe"; "Maybe I am deserving of love"; "What kind of connection do I have to all things? What is my deepest nature . . . my real self?"

Expanding the moment or eliciting the bigger picture provides a container that is sustaining and profound. We may be inclined to learn emotion regulation skills because they will help us live more effectively and feel less victimized by waves of emotions and thoughts. There may, however, be slippage with this pragmatic motivational base. Providing extra fuel to the intention to practice these skills may be the aspiration to walk a meaningful and admirable path—and for some, to walk the path that God wishes that she or he walk.

In addition to fueling intention, *expand-the-moment* contemplation concretely enhances emotional regulation. I breathe deeply and connect to the universe or God's world. The rage or despair is held in a larger container where inevitably all is okay. As a result, the incident provoking the arising emotion seems a bit smaller and less significant. Perhaps I may sense the compassion that my higher power, the universe, or God has for me, and the ensuing serenity or experience of the thread of love that weaves through creation allows me to let go of my constricted, vengeful state.

For some, this connection is the glimpse of the spiritual world that is available. The call is to move out of our small self where we tend to view the story of the world. *Here I am walking through the world. This is what is happening to me. This is what I like and don't like. These are the people I see and come in contact with and what I think about them. I wish that person liked me more . . . I really don't care whether that person likes me or not because I don't really like that person very much . . . I am worried about whether I am making enough money . . . Maybe I will have more in a few years . . . I think I would look better if I lost a few pounds . . . I hate how much everyone cares about how you look . . . Maybe I will go on a diet . . . I am kinda lazy . . . I need to work harder . . . Maybe my life will never be satisfying . . . I am feeling blue . . . I need to just lie down . . . There I go being lazy again. . . .*

Touching the spiritual world—whatever form that may take—helps us touch a picture that is bigger than this quality of small self. When the container for the kind of rumination depicted (rumination is a fundamental ingredient in depression; see Strosahl & Robinson, 2008) is larger than the small self, the content of the rumination is less compelling and the individual is able to attain a bird's-eye view that puts these worries into perspective.

Ultimately, the task of emotion regulation is about feeling settled in a world that is fundamentally unsettled—that is to say, always changing. Discrete emotion regulation skills may improve the thermostat's efficiency to ascertain and fine-tune emotional distress and expression. This approach rests in the mastery of skills, an unsettling process for people who have struggled often in life, in order to feel stable. Leaning on spirituality may help with the larger view that settled or unsettled, you are still loved, you still belong, you are still valuable, and there is still some point in which to rest and seek refuge. Relax and take a breath!

Validation and Acceptance to Support Client Change

We return to the primary dialectic of DBT-WR presented in Chapter 1. For clients to develop confidence in nonreactively being with and responding to arising situations, thoughts, and emotions, they need to experience a calm and accepting holding environment within the clinical or service context. This kind of environment may run counter to the life experience of many of our clients—the very experiences that contributed to emotion regulation challenges:

> Pervasive invalidation occurs when, more often than not, caregivers treat our valid primary responses as incorrect, inaccurate, inappropriate, pathological, or not to be taken seriously. Primary responses of interest are persistently squelched or mocked; normal needs for soothing are regularly neglected or shamed; honest motives consistently doubted and misinterpreted. The person therefore learns to avoid, interrupt, and control his or her own natural inclinations and primary emotional response. Like a creature in a chamber with an electrified grid on

the floor, he or she learns to avoid any step that results in pain and invalidation. (Koerner, 2012, p. 6)

Many clients do experience the world as invalidating and hurtful. They may enter interactions with a service provider on guard for potential provider responses that may cause harm and their repertoire vis-à-vis a provider or clinician may mirror their repertoire in other parts of life. Challenging circumstances, such as developing a relationship with a clinician, may elicit fight, flight, or freeze responses or, at least, provoke some degree of fear, reluctance, and reactivity.

Clinicians and practitioners really do "hold the cards" with clients. Clients are expected to be revealing and risk taking and are not sure what to expect back from practitioners. By virtue of their client status, they are "one down"—the crazy one, the one who is in trouble, the one who is unstable, and the one who is in need of help. (These issues may be accentuated with mandated clients.) They know little about the degree to which clinicians, in their personal lives, experience any of these issues, and clients are not even sure if they want to know. In the face of these dynamics, clients do what they can to protect themselves. Emotionally activated by the therapy or helping context, they may reactively and not so skillfully respond. After all, they are working with the limited skills that make them candidates for DBT-WR in the first place. There are particular elements to consider regarding the helping context's influence on reactivity.

First, clients may not know how activated and fearful they are about the power differential, expected intimacy and vulnerability, and limit setting embedded in the practitioner–client relationship. Because they lack the requisite mindfulness skills to tune into their experience and to spot their primary emotions—skills they will eventually learn in DBT-WR—they may reactively manifest anger, avoidance, or judgmentalism to ward off their painful feelings.

Second, many clients have a trauma background. Regardless of the effectiveness of the practitioner–client relationship, people may struggle revealing parts of themselves because of the shame and humiliation involved; in other words, the relationship does not feel safe (these dynamics will be explored further in Chapter 4). Denial, minimization, defensiveness, and even hostility may be the alternatives that seem the best or, at least, most available given the client's perception that she or he is under threat in the service context.

Third, the clinician or service provider response may enhance the degree to which the environment is experienced as nonvalidating and, perhaps, unsafe. Clinicians may react to client walls, barriers, and emotional displays with our own set of responses that are not necessarily skillful. If not particularly tuned into the client's own process or reasons for reluctantly engaging with us, we may emotionally react with labeling the client as "resistant," "manipulative," "inappropriate," or "noncompliant." As we go down the road of dismissing or subtly rejecting the client, perhaps with a hint of anger or frustration, we have entered the client–practitioner reactivity dance.

The practitioner's relentless focus on client acceptance is fundamental to effective DBT-WR. Acceptance of the client's process provides a model for the client's own acceptance of her or his internal life. The clinical task is to help clients radically accept or come to terms with what arises for them. This acceptance allows for the client to be okay in the moment and move to a nonreactive choice about how to respond. Not only does acceptance facilitate the client's coming to terms with her or his own experience, it provides direction for the response choice. In other words, the person who experiences acceptance may be the person who moves toward responses that reflect self-care and self-compassion. This situation precisely describes the dialectic between acceptance and change. People sense that their authentic selves are accepted; they integrate that experience so that they can more effectively accept their own authentic

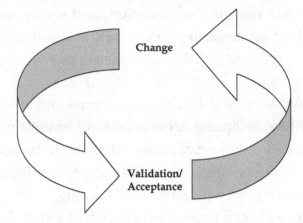

Figure 2.3 Acceptance and Change Dialectic

selves; their responses and behaviors change, in that they are less reactive, more skillful, and life promoting; their enhanced efficacy and positive feedback from the larger society enhances their sense of acceptance. Figure 2.3 pictorially depicts the acceptance and change dialectic.

Example of Nonvalidating Responses

Radical acceptance in the clinical context emerges from the practitioner's life practice and resultant conscious use-of-self. The interface of radical acceptance and the clinical use-of-self is covered in Chapter 5. What is primarily important is the clinician's intention to truly accept the client for who he or she is and to maintain awareness of this intention even as challenges arise with the relationship or as clinician judgments arise.

The client experiences radical acceptance from the professional through observing and interacting with the practitioner's open, accepting, nonjudgmental stance, which may be psychologically and spiritually based, as well as through receiving validating comments. However, our radically accepting stance may be compromised when we are irritated with a client because of the individual's characteristics or behavior, lack of progress, or lack of appreciation for our professional efforts. When judgments, emotional distance, and impatience override empathy, compassion, and appreciation, our sense of celebration regarding *this person* is diminished, and the client will experience that the environment is not unconditionally accepting.

A dearth of validating comments may also contribute to the client experiencing a nonaccepting environment. Of course, if there is limited practitioner intention to be accepting and there are elements interfering with acceptance, then genuine validating comments will not be forthcoming.

The client's limited experience of validation may also come from the practitioner's overreliance and hyperfocus on content. Recently, I was going through a DBT-WR lesson and a group member was clearly struggling. Her mouth was in pain from tooth and gum damage caused by long-term methamphetamine use, and she was dreading the upcoming intervention, the only one available for many poor people—getting her teeth pulled. In an attempt to tie her experience back to mindfulness possibilities, I discussed themes that Jon Kabat-Zinn (1990) has raised in MBSR, such as staying in the present, being with the breath, and letting go of stories related to the pain (e.g., stories regarding how long the pain has been going on, as well as constructed scenarios about the future). Practicing this way, I reasoned would help her during the group.

As I reflected later on the group, I realized that my approach made her invisible and did not validate her actual experience of pain, as well as the courage and determination she had demonstrated in showing up that day and in not taking a narcotic pain reliever. In some way, I had not taken her experience seriously and focused on doling out advice and taking advantage of the available "teaching moment." Her lack of appreciation for my intervention was apparent. I mended fences the next week and apologized for my lack of sensitivity. I thought it was important for clients to see that, though I had been insensitive and nonvalidating, I could still give them the message that they deserved more than what I provided on that day. I asked for their forgiveness, though I would understand if they were reluctant.

Other practitioner infractions related to invalidation are more subtle. Clients are "extremely sensitive to all cues that might bring the painful zap of invalidation" (Koerner, 2012, p. 7). Challenging caregiving relationships, stigmatized group membership, emotionally reactive personal proclivities, and unresponsive and demeaning systems all set the stage for and perpetuate the client's experience of invalidation. In order to reverse the cycle, we start with deliberate and intentional acceptance and validation to set the stage for emotion regulation and client fulfillment and happiness.

Three

Applying DBT to Mental Health and Substance Abuse Recovery

Overview of Issues

Recovery has different meanings in the substance abuse world and the mental health arena. This divergence stems from and, in turn, contributes to service delivery systems that often have conflicting aims and leave people with dual diagnosis challenges largely underserved (Burnam & Watkins, 2006; Minkoff & Cline, 2006; Sterling, Chi, & Hinman, 2011). This chapter will examine the philosophical underpinnings of mental health recovery and substance abuse recovery, and will outline issues for people who are considered as having a "dual diagnosis."

The Substance Abuse and Mental Health Services Administration (SAMHSA) has attempted to reach a unifying definition to clear confusion regarding the term *recovery*. They state that

> Recovery from mental disorders and/or substance use disorders . . . [is a] process of change through which individuals improve their health and wellness, live a self-directed life, and strive to reach their full potential. (SAMHSA, 2012)

The SAMHSA (2012) explication notes that there are four areas of focus or "dimensions" that are relevant for making progress on the recovery path: health, home, purpose, and community. There is flexibility within these dimensions because of their caution to not impose a cookie-cutter image about what recovery is supposed to look like. Instead, the guiding recovery principles include "recovery is person-driven" and "recovery occurs via many pathways."

When specifically addressing substance abuse, however, the flexible, person-centered approach directed toward mental health recovery is dropped, and the explicit statement, "abstaining from use of alcohol, illicit drugs, and nonprescribed medications if one has an addiction problem" appears (SAMHSA, 2012). Later in the document, the precise course for substance abuse recovery is declared within the overall (mental health and substance abuse) rubric of recovery:

> Abstinence from the use of alcohol, illicit drugs, and non-prescribed medications is the goal for those with addictions. Use of tobacco and non-prescribed or illicit drugs is not safe for anyone. (SAMHSA, 2012)

Although an initial intent of the document was to unify the definition of recovery, the orientation, interestingly, shifts when drug/alcohol abuse is involved.

Other elements within SAMHSA's (2012) statement would likely be embraced by clients or consumers who struggle with mental health issues, substance abuse issues, or both:

➤ Recovery emerges from hope.

➤ Recovery is person driven.

➤ Recovery occurs via many pathways.

➤ Recovery is holistic.

➤ Recovery is supported by peers and allies.

➤ Recovery is supported through relationship and social networks.

➤ Recovery is culturally based and influenced.

➤ Recovery is supported by addressing trauma.

➤ Recovery involves individual, family, and community strengths and responsibility.

➤ Recovery is based on respect.

For the most part, the development and emergence of these guiding principles reflects the political and treatment demands of people in the mental health recovery movement (see Davidson et al., 2009; Slade, 2009; Walsh, 2013). Mental health recovery proponents have challenged institutions and social structures around (a) the usual ways of conducting business (e.g., stigmatizing, overrelying on medication, discounting client voice), (b) the paradigms that undergird professional approaches and methods (e.g., expert driven, one size fits all), and (c) the levels of respect with which clients or consumers are generally treated (e.g., infantilized, hyperfocused on compliance).

Thus, as we examine the application of dialectical behavior therapy or dialectical behavior therapy for wellness and recovery (DBT-WR) across settings, we need to not only address the clinical implications of this work according to diagnosed disorders (see Dimeff & Koerner, 2007), but *we also need to take into account and assure that the practitioner–client container for practice incorporates mental health recovery principles designed to promote client empowerment and wellness.*

Practicing Mental Health Recovery in DBT-WR

The recovery community has raised a number of objections regarding traditional mental health delivery. Treatment models conventionally proceed from the supposition that there is an explanatory model for understanding the experience of the "disordered" individual. In fact, the more that we know about the client—his or her diagnosis; patterns of dysfunction; or, in the case of DBT-WR, the nature and degree to which he or she struggles with emotion regulation—the more we can hone in on using a precise set of interventions designed to counteract the person's dysfunctions. The recovery movement, however, identifies that "it is dangerous to impose a model of understanding the (client's) experience, rather than supporting the person to find their own interpretation" (Slade, 2009, p. 28).

A recent DBT-WR group interaction shed light on the value of honoring the client's personal beliefs about what is helpful. I was discussing with the group the importance of *noticing* our negative self-judgments rather than attempting reflexively to replace them with positive or affirming statements. As mentioned earlier in the book, thought replacement is a cognitive strategy that may have some merit, but as Linehan suggests, the practice keeps one locked into the process of judging. In other words, the practice of changing "I am bad" into "I am good" may have some merit, but, in doing so, one essentially *practices* judgment and counterjudgment every time this kind of cognitive strategy is utilized. The mindfulness-oriented approach is to notice the judgment, describe it, and radically accept that the judgment has arisen. The capacity of being an observer to judgment leads to an enhanced capacity for not believing thoughts and for seeing thoughts just as they are—thoughts rather than truths. Engaging in this more mindful, DBT-oriented practice leads to developing additional skills such as *defusion*, or the releasing of the influence that arising thoughts and emotions would have on one's overall well-being.

One group member was "not having" my elegant description about how to dispassionately observe negative self-judgments. She stated emphatically that she "just does not go there." Her life had been so much about negativity that she was not going to make any place for that stuff and she was going to focus *only* on the positive. When I asked whether any negative thoughts still sometimes came, she wondered aloud whether I was *trying* to inject negativity with my question. She insisted, perhaps in accord with 12-step ideas about "stinkin thinkin," that the best approach was to rid herself of negativity and not make any space for it.

In essence, the client rejected the paradigm concerning a mindfulness approach to negative self-judgments or statements. I validated and radically accepted her view regarding the proposed mindfulness-based approach, not so much because I thought arguing with her perspective would not be constructive, but because of my commitment to maintain a mental health recovery stance. Not only does this client have the "right" to declare what is helpful or not helpful for her, but there is extraordinary value in the practitioner's understanding, learning from, and collaborating with the client's own perspective about what help looks like, or what has been called the "client's theory of change" (Duncan & Miller, 2000; Duncan, Miller, & Sparks, 2004).

This kind of listening and collaboration helps practitioners transcend the "one-size-fits-all" mentality that sometimes deprives evidence-based practices of immediate relevance and individual responsiveness. In other words, it is not enough to say, in the case of DBT or DBT-WR, that this person or these persons have emotion regulation challenges, and here is the treatment package they *need* in order to address their challenges.

However, highly idiographic or anecdotally driven practice elevates clinician whim or perpetual reinvention as preferred practice and inevitably falls short as recovery-oriented practice (Slade, 2009). *Therefore, the dialectical synthesis is desirable of, on the one hand, evidence-based or supported practices while, on the other hand, a practice orientation of collaboratively arriving at meaning and transcending the disempowering expert–nonexpert dichotomy.*

This dialectical synthesis is similar to DBT-WR's central dialectic discussed in Chapter 1—moving beyond the superficial understanding of validation and change as apparent opposites. With DBT-WR, we come to realize that, although we can choose in a given moment to focus on either validation or change, there is a possibility for synthesis and that validation/acceptance and change may reinforce each other. Similarly, we realize the limitations of leaning solely in the direction of *either* practice model fidelity and uniformity *or* individualized, atheoretical spontaneity. A synthesis is required involving a theoretically sound and tested structure for help with a simultaneous deep respect for individual client meanings, aspirations, voices, and feedback within the treatment context. The respect for the individual's nuanced process and aspirations reflects a definition of recovery that is commonly cited (Anthony, 1993):

> Recovery is a deeply personal, unique process of changing one's attitudes, values, feelings, goals, skills, and/or roles. It is a way of living a satisfying, hopeful, and contributing life even within the limitations caused by illness. Recovery involves the development of new meaning and purpose in one's life as one grows beyond the (sometimes) catastrophic effects of mental illness. (Slade, 2009, p. 38)

Thus, within this book's DBT-WR structure that has supportive evidence involving mindfulness attainment for dual diagnosis clients (Richards & Sehr, 2011), the client who says "this doesn't work for me" is honored and her perspective is considered as *personal wisdom*. There may be a temptation, in one way or another, to discount her view; with the clinical thinking: "*After all, she is just a 'patient' with emotion regulation challenges—what does she know about how to deal with her struggles?*

If she were so good at knowing how to respond in the world, she wouldn't be having the problems that she has. On the other hand, I (the professional) am armed with scientific knowledge and tools. If she were just less resistant she would be better able to take advantage of the clinical process. It's her own pathology and/or lack of understanding that is getting in the way of her making progress."

The encouragement here is to drop this familiar clinical narrative and to incorporate recovery-oriented thinking into DBT-WR. The first part of the mental health recovery approach emphasizes the quality of the consumer–practitioner relationship as key for positive mental health outcomes (Slade, 2009; Davidson et al., 2009; Walsh, 2013). This emphasis is in accord with evidence that connects positive therapeutic outcomes to the strength and viability of the therapeutic relationship (Bertolino & Miller, 2012; Duncan et al., 2004; Duncan, Miller, Wampold, & Hubble, 2010; Hewitt & Coffey, 2005; Norcross & Wampold, 2011). One element of a positive relationship involves the practitioner's willingness to account for and adapt to the nuanced thinking, aspirations, life situations, and personal qualities and strengths of particular clients. Norcross and Wampold's (2011) meta-analysis of studies related to evidence-based practice led to the conclusion that "adapting or tailoring the therapy relationship to specific consumer characteristics enhances the effectiveness of treatment" (Walsh, 2013).

In addition to a recovery emphasis on practitioner–client relationship quality, the second facet of recovery-oriented thinking within DBT-WR relates to, as mentioned, the honoring of the client's point of view and perspective. One consumer activist, Arana Pearson, recommends that clients even the status playing field with practitioners through use of the initials QBE after their names—"qualified by experience" (Slade, 2009). Again, we enter an interesting dialectic. Practitioners have formalized practice knowledge, a diagnostic framework that perhaps enhances understanding of the challenges that clients face, a set of curriculum or practice tools that may help establish a structure leading to positive results, and ideas about relationship structure (e.g., attendance, rules, boundaries). Clients, however, have opinions and feelings about practitioner methods, have aspirations to participate on some level in their own treatment, have wisdom about previous personal efforts or new practitioner proposed techniques that may or may not be effective, have inclinations based on their own readiness for change (see DiClemente, 2006), and have an image of the kind of connection they would like to have with the practitioner.

Operationalizing this dialectic may involve practitioner creativity or flexibility to step outside the structure and consult with a client regarding how to proceed. While discussing the skill opposite action, for example, one young man proudly talked about the level of progress he was making. He mentioned that his mother had not been acknowledging his progress, and instead continued to emphasize his shortcomings. Rather than indulging in my own (as therapist) reactivity concerning his mother's actions, I asked the client about whether he wished to abandon the DBT-WR lesson for the day so that his mother would come into the session. I personally had no agenda to head in either direction (the planned DBT-WR lesson versus the family session). The client chose to discuss critically important issues with the family and did so quite skillfully.

A recovery orientation contributed to the session's process, direction, and result. First, I willingly dropped my agenda for the session because I deliberately work within the dialectic between structure and responsiveness. Responsiveness in the moment builds client faith that the structure is not arbitrarily adhered to and that immediate needs count. Responsibly parting from the structure, if done thoughtfully and in balance, *validates* the client's reality and models for clients that situations can arise and receive skillful attention and responses. In fact, it is a kind of *opposite action* on behalf of the clinician to let go of the day's lesson and allow for the possibility that the session will take a different direction. Another clinician approach would be to emotionally react to a change in the agenda or not accept that change may have a potential benefit.

Second, the client had a choice about how to proceed. A collaborative treatment environment places responsibility for the client's personal well-being in his or her lap and communicates, "This is your time here; I want to follow your wisdom about what would be the best use of this time." Respect for client decision making is conveyed, and the client may have more investment in the process and result of the conversation than had I said, "We should have your mom come in and address these issues together" or "Let's set aside what is happening at home and continue with the planned lesson for today." Making space for client choice is empowering for clients and flattens the hierarchy.

The model of "I know what is best for you so I will control how we will proceed" inevitably reinforces that the client's well-being is a professional matter. Slade (2009) characterizes that in the clinical model of mental health, expertise resides in the professional and treatment is deemed as necessary and appropriate. In recovery-oriented practice, *expertise* is either shared (between the consumer and practitioner) or predominantly resides in the consumer.

Third, I normalized the dilemmas of parties throughout the family conversation, so as to reduce blaming and pathologizing and to enhance understanding, personal validation, and interpersonal acceptance. Although maintaining the structure of mutual reflective listening, I placed my hope in the capacity of the mother–son dyad to learn what they needed to do to move forward. Sometimes I shared my perceptions of some of their dynamics and offered that I was not sure—which was no lie—about how they would emerge from their struggles. They offered ideas, sometimes based on the DBT-WR lessons that we had previously covered.

When the practitioner accepts and works within the illustrated dialectic, she concurrently holds boundaries, coherent methodologies, and treatment structure on the one hand, while honoring the client's view, adapting to individualized needs, and accounting for client strengths and aspirations on the other. Paradoxically, in a collaborative framework, boundaries may be more effectively realized, because rules and norms do not seem arbitrarily and insensitively imposed. Similarly, a collaborative framework may induce more buy-in regarding the overall treatment because acceptance and consideration of the client's nuanced view and input regarding the therapy context empowers and encourages the client to move forward and take responsibility for wellness.

Although a proponent of the recovery movement, Dr. Frederick Frese, a researcher, professor, high-level mental health administrator, and mental health consumer with paranoid schizophrenia, believes that there needs to be a continuum regarding recovery-oriented practice. When people are severely impaired, the language of "self-determination" is not so relevant because these individuals may be in the grips of their mental illness (Frese, 2013; Frese, Stanley, Kress, & Vogel-Scibilia, 2001). Applying the language of dialectics, we can see where high structure and directed practitioner involvement may create more opportunities to advance "self-determination" than placing a lot of decision making and responsibility in the hands of a person deeply suffering with psychosis and/or anxiety.

> For persons who are so seriously impaired in decision making capacity that they are incapable of determining what is in their best interest, a paternalistic, externally reasoned treatment approach would seem to be not only appropriate, but also necessary, for the well being of the impaired individual. However, as these impaired persons begin to benefit from externally initiated interventions, the locus of control should increasingly shift from treatment provider to the person who is recovering. As individuals recover, they must gradually be afforded a

larger role in the selection of treatments and services. Throughout the recovery process, persons should be given maximal opportunity to regain control over their lives. (Frese et al., 2001, p. 1463)

The dialectic of treatment structure and individual self-expression establishes the ground for the client's work on enhancing discipline and fulfilling treatment responsibilities on the one hand and the assertion of individuality and personal decision making on the other. Once again, the apparent opposites—structure and individualism—work hand-in-hand reinforcing one another. The DBT-WR *structure* provides a safe, reliable practice container facilitating the client to make the *individual decision* to skillfully respond in the middle of arising, intense emotions. The structure as well as occasional practitioner directedness may also help establish a bottom-line level of functioning so that the consumer may have the capacity to make meaningful decisions. At the same time, the individual, *self-determined* intention of moving forward and creating a life worth living leads the client to lean on the *structure* of DBT-WR exercises, lessons, and explanatory schema. In traditional mental health practice, the starting point of this explanatory schema begins with a mental health diagnosis.

Recovery Critique of Deficit-Based Diagnosis

A mental health diagnosis is frequently a powerful lens through which to view an individual. There are certainly benefits of diagnosis, but, on the detrimental side, the labeling process may enhance the person's experienced stigma while devaluing the nuanced parts of the person's life such as resilience, hope, strategies for living, contributions to others, and strengths. Unfortunately, the diagnosis may also bias practitioners regarding the potential growth trajectory of the client as well as the practitioner's belief that professional help and direction is "required" for client progress and well-being.

A danger of a deficit-based diagnosis is that it may spawn negativity or water the seeds of aversion toward identified individuals. Clinicians may act out their aversion and accompanying lack of empathic connection through authoritarian behavior. Clients with a borderline personality disorder diagnosis, for example, are sometimes vulnerable because of derisive professional thinking. Combining minimally empathic and objectifying helper behavior with a crisis environment, such as a psychiatric hospital unit, create some scenarios that are unsatisfactory. A hospital-based psychiatrist threatening mentally ill clients—"You will not leave the hospital until you do as I say," or refusing to provide a prescription at discharge for medications because the psychiatrist is upset that the client made an independent, "against medical advice," decision to leave the hospital—pits professional against patient. This kind of disrespectful behavior may, in part, rest on the belief that people with mental illness or mental health challenges are less than fully human. The categorization of people by "illness" may perpetuate oppressive practice and the placement of clients or patients in deviant, incompetent roles (Rapp & Goscha, 2006).

Once a person is seen as "a borderline," "a meth addict," or "a schizophrenic" the clinician may be disposed to "treat" the malady, which means administer some kind of intervention to a passive recipient. In a traditional paradigm, the main task of the ill recipient is to comply with or adhere to the crafted treatment package. The lens of illness sometimes

> supports the belief that the clinician's job is to treat the illness, not the person's job to recover their life. It fosters dependency—the good patient is compliant with treatment. (Slade, 2009, p. 23)

Recovery-oriented practice has a critical view of the "good patient" or "good client" construct. Whether mandated or not, practitioners may be inclined to equate positive client work with how much clients are aligning with the rules, norms, and philosophies of the treatment context. This mentality leads to reduced empathy for clients who may question the practitioner's methods or expertise, or penalizing clients whose personal challenges make it difficult for them to comply with attendance policies or other treatment standards.

Becoming Closer to Normal

The reason that traditional mental health practices may focus in the direction of client compliance derives from the belief that treatment is ultimately in the service of minimizing the "oddness" of the individual and making her or him the most normal she or he could be. The practitioner's overemphasis on monitoring and enforcing client or consumer adherence to a medication regimen reduces the priority on accounting for client/consumer aspirations, resilience, and hope. An elevated focus on behavioral markers approximating socially acceptable standards similarly leans practitioners in the direction of aligning with social standards related to enforcing normalcy.

This discussion is not meant to romanticize unchecked mental illness. People who are struggling may do better if their minds and behaviors are more settled (e.g., their moods are not so variable and/or debilitating, their behavior is not causing community or personal suffering, hallucinations are not so frequent or intense, emotional reactivity is reduced). Suffering for clients and for surrounding family and community members may also be ameliorated if, in fact, the person becomes "more stable" or starts thinking, feeling, and acting more like the "average person." Sometimes from good intentions, practitioners would like to wipe away the pain-producing dysfunction and make change happen. Amidst our frustration about how difficult or complicated it is to accomplish this, we may be inclined to compromise the client's self-determination and "push them" to respond in the way that we believe is most constructive.

Proponents of mental health recovery believe that if practitioners try to take over the lives of their clients in the name of making positive things happen, a few negative results occur: the client experiences less respect, the client receives a message that positive results are controlled by professional reasoning and strategizing, the client's own strategies for coping and personal wisdom are devalued, the client's aspirations and wishes transcending simple symptom management become unseen, the client's life is reduced to managing symptoms endemic to whatever illness the client is diagnosed with.

Patricia Deegan, PhD, a mental health consumer and one of the most eloquent voices for mental health recovery, addressed the issues outlined earlier. She asserted that a major recovery principle is that "People can move from just *taking* medications to *using* them as part of their own recovery process" (Deegan, 1995, p. 1). In another publication outlining her personal recovery process, Deegan discusses the spiritual and philosophical task at hand for people struggling with mental illness:

> The goal of the recovery process is *not* to become normal. The goal is to embrace our human vocation of becoming more deeply, more fully human. The goal is not normalization. The goal is to become the unique, awesome, never to be repeated human being that we are called to be. The philosopher Martin Heidegger said that to be human means to be a question in search of an answer. Those of us who have been labeled with mental illness are not de facto excused from this most fundamental task of becoming human. In fact because many of us have experienced our lives and dreams shattering in the wake of mental illness, one of the most essential challenges that faces us is to ask, "who can I become and why should I say 'yes' to life?" (Deegan, 2001, p. 3; italics mine)

Responsive DBT-WR attempts to capture the spirit of these words. A danger in teaching skills to clients is the potential establishment of expert and nonexpert roles. Clients may be viewed through the lens of their emotion regulation deficits, and we may envision our task as helping people get more in line with what healthy emotion regulation is supposed to look like. This orientation emerges, not so much because clinicians are not respectful enough, but because it has merit. Clients *do* have emotion regulation challenges that contribute to dramatic consequences in their lives as well as to enhanced suffering. This suffering is reduced when emotion regulation capacity is improved. Furthermore, clients deeply appreciate these lessons and talk about how they have saved their lives (see Van Gelder, 2010, for a profound personal account of DBT's role in helping her reclaim her life). Patricia Deegan and others, however, call for a balance in perspectives. See the individual or the group member for their "awesomeness"; appreciate their wisdom and strengths (see Frese, 2013; Saleebey, 2012); be aware of the stigmatizing use of labels; account for the way in which the clinical position, service structures, or practitioner behavior activates raw, often traumatized clients; and work diligently to be respectful, appreciative, and nonreactive.

Mental health recovery pushes practitioners to question the utility of time-honored practices, to remain open to various possibilities, and to move out from behind the rigid hierarchy that sometimes divides clinician and client. When a client challenges a practitioner, for example, it is the practitioner's job to not get defensive, not take the challenge personally, and respond in a congruent manner that, in fact, models for the client that conflict and doubt is acceptable and can be contained and effectively addressed. Rather than clinically assessing this kind of behavior as indicative of denial, resistance, or defiance, there are normalizing and strengths-oriented frames that are possible.

In recovery-oriented practice, we appreciate the complexity and contradictions of the client–practitioner relationship. On a certain level our funding sources—whether government entities, family members, or insurance companies—appreciate the practitioner's having influence regarding the client's level of stability or "deviant" behavior. The recovery movement meanwhile challenges us that *externally imposed goals regarding mental stability:*

➤ Compromise the ethical principle of client self-determination.

➤ Reduce the struggling person's life to a collection of symptoms.

➤ Simplify intervention strategies often emphasizing medication "management."

➤ Fuel the unwise and illusory notion that the professionals are capable of simplistically controlling client behavior.

➤ Lead to demeaning mental health practice.

Are They More Normal Yet?

Another element regarding clinical-oriented assessment and diagnosis is that "professionals don't see people as often when they are coping" (Slade, 2009, p. 152), thus the practitioner's view about who clients are and how they live is skewed. In the previously discussed example involving the woman's critiquing the group exercise, we may be disposed to assume she is in need of expert opinion and guidance; after all, the criminal justice system is mandating that she be in treatment so, logically, it would seem, she has little to offer in the way of positive coping strategies and perspectives on emotion regulation.

Professional blind spots fuel the mental health recovery movement's demand that the consumer's (or the word "survivor" is sometimes used, see Deegan, 1995) voice is heard and respected, that self-determination is maximized, that the hierarchy be flattened, and that the treatment process involve collaboration, mutual discovery, and sharing of knowledge. One demand from the mental health recovery community is congruent with this view:

> In the process of evaluation, treatment, and rehabilitation, recovery-oriented practitioners [need to] therefore place as much, or possibly even more, emphasis on their clients' personal narratives and goals as they do on their clients' symptoms, deficits and diagnosis. (Davidson et al., 2009, p. 22)

Recovery-Oriented Relationships With Practitioners

Interestingly, SAMHSA's (2012) statement on recovery mentioned that "recovery is supported by addressing trauma." We will explore trauma in more detail later; for now it is important to note that many clients have a trauma history. For example, women who have a substance abuse diagnosis have a PTSD diagnosis between 30% and 59% of the time (Najavits, 2002). Trauma is pervasive among people with mental illness, and the restrictive PTSD diagnostic parameters—only considering direct personal experience of situations "involving actual or threatened death or serious injury" along with sexual abuse— does not fully account for the degree of psychological trauma suffered (Briere & Scott, 2006). People experiencing collective community trauma (see the Satsuki Ina, 1999, exploration of ethnic group trauma in *Children of the Camps*), trauma from dealing with mental illness, trauma from being consistently humiliated while living in physically and emotionally compromised situations are not eligible, based on these situations alone, for a PTSD diagnosis. It is projected that the PTSD definition in the *Diagnostic and Statistical Manual of Mental Disorders* fifth edition (*DSM-V*) will not enhance inclusivity or increase the overall frequency of the diagnosis (United States Department of Veterans Affairs, National Center for PTSD, 2012).

Trauma is mentioned vis-à-vis the practitioner–client relationship because many of our trauma-surviving clients are activated in sessions with us. If we are committed to recovery, we must not only work toward creating a respectful, collaborative relationship accounting for the well-rounded aspirations and hopes of our clients, we need to—as SAMHSA (2012) says—"address" trauma, and in this case trauma's role within the client–practitioner relationship. Accounting for trauma within the client–practitioner relationship means becoming aware of how clients may engage in fight–freeze–flight behavior in the clinical context. There are a number of factors or triggers that may precipitate this response.

First, engagement with clients sometimes is overly invasive. Clients may be highly activated as they report on events that have happened in their lives, and the holding environment may not be sufficiently mature to contain the intensity of people's circumstances and accompanying feelings. Some people disassociate as they talk about various situations, or they reexperience rather than therapeutically integrate the trauma (Briere & Scott, 2006; Herman, 1997; Miller-Karas & Leitch, 2009). Strategies for titrating (Briere & Scott, 2006), assisting in constructing narratives (Mollica, 2006), or enhancing safety or resources (Miller-Karas & Leitch, 2009; Najavits, 2002) will be mentioned further in the next chapter.

Second, engagement with professionals, especially in "high-stakes," mandated situations, leads to power dynamics that are reminiscent of victimization experiences because the holders of power may be experienced as unkind and not understanding. If a client with a substantial number of previous absences is genuinely sick within a mandated substance abuse program, she may come to believe that the hard line being taken with her is based on the practitioner's lack of kindness and understanding. Although the practitioner may argue that the client's past pattern of less responsible absences set up the current situation, the client experiences that her current, legitimate illness leads to her having to make a lose-lose decision. She will face either having to go to a treatment group while sick or face as—she perceives it—an unforgiving, arbitrary, uncaring clinician, probation officer, and criminal justice system that may—in her view—punish her for being sick. If she honors her body and stays home, her noncompliance may be highlighted by the system. She will not be validated for how much she loves her children, how much she is struggling with her present illness, nor what kind of horrific history that she has had to endure.

Building relationships with recovery principles demands that we recognize and have empathy for just what clients are up against. Recovery does not imply a certain degree of leniency or an abandonment of structure and clarity. Sometimes a recovery-oriented relationship involves the practitioner's moving beyond the conventional methods of blanket rule enforcement, standard lectures, or expectations of client sharing that do not feel safe given the strength of the professional relationship. We radically accept that our presence may be provocative and we aim—at the very least—to do no harm. Most thankfully, many clients are resilient and will look for evidence of our caring and fairness. They will find ways to engage even though we could have done more to account for their trauma history.

Respect for Clients Within DBT-WR

Dialectical behavior therapy was designed to work with people diagnosed with borderline personality disorder. Respect was embedded in the theoretical model, in that acceptance and validation were emphasized. Additionally, the DBT treatment outcome pointed to helping clients construct "a life worth living" despite the treatment context often involving "unrelenting crises and management of high-risk suicidal behavior" (Koerner & Dimeff, 2007, p. 1).

Asking clients to speak on behalf of their Wise Minds is a way in which DBT therapists attempt to tap into individualized client coping styles and wisdom regarding challenging circumstances (Koerner, 2012). This form of inquiry differs from the practitioner generating prescriptive alternatives.

DBT also emphasizes practitioner authenticity, which incorporates a client's concern about the therapeutic process. Under the technique "extending," the practitioner takes a client's concern to the logical conclusion. Some clients may assume that their voice may not be considered while they are, let's say, making a vague complaint about the therapeutic process. One response by a DBT therapist may be:

> If this therapy isn't helping, then we need to do something about that. Do you think you should fire me? This is very serious. (Koerner, 2012, p. 156)

This kind of response integrates the use-of-self styles that are part of the DBT or DBT-WR practitioner's repertoire. Practitioners are encouraged to be *reciprocal*, including "self-disclosure, warm engagement, and genuineness to answer [a] question" that a client may ask (Koerner, 2012, p. 148). There is also permission to respectfully set limits, to talk about how a client's behavior may affect the practitioner, and to find ways to establish intimacy. Citing Tsai et al. (2008), Koerner (2012) asserts that the DBT practitioner seeks to create a relationship that is similar to a congruent, fulfilling connection that one may establish outside the therapy setting.

Within the *reciprocal* style, the practitioner may address the difficult challenges related to boundaries. We can normalize the confusion that sometimes comes with this relationship; it is challenging. We may say, "Sometimes the relationship feels so intimate, yet we (the client and practitioner) do not spend time together outside of the office. We care about each other, we mean a lot to each other; this relationship is difficult to figure out." In this response, our heart goes out to the client grappling with understanding boundaries. We truly understand the dilemma, and when we say it is "hard to figure out" we mean, on some level, that it is hard for both of us. We do not make the client wrong for struggling or misunderstanding, and we ultimately validate the client and what she or he means to us.

While the reciprocal style promotes acceptance/validation, the *irreverent* style is usually directed to the change part of the dialectic. Irreverence offers different opportunities for confrontation and may help wake the client from a fixed or stuck place (Koerner, 2012). In a recent interaction, I spoke with a sometimes angry and skeptical client and called her the "star" of the group. This comment changed her frame regarding her place in the group—she had assumed I was frustrated with her and did not appreciate her participation. Calling her a star also changed the way that clients viewed involvement in the group—you don't have to either agree with the leader or keep your mouth shut in order to be appreciated. Irreverence directed toward change ultimately related back to acceptance. The irreverent communication conveyed that you can show up to the group as yourself and you will be loved and supported. Calling her "the star" was irreverent because it shook group members from the familiar ground of "everyone here is thought of equally." For the individual called "star," whatever rebellious or troublemaker role she imagined settling into was no longer available; her comments were contributing to the group's growth, and I was clearly enjoying her presence.

Caution needs to be exercised when utilizing irreverent communication. First, the practitioner needs to be aware of personal intentions so as to not vent sarcastically under the guise of being irreverent. Effective irreverence needs to emerge from a centered and nonreactive practitioner. Second, what some may experience as helpful, humorous, and memorable banter, others may experience as insensitive, uncaring, mocking, or insulting. From a recovery perspective, we do all we can to tune into the strength and trust of the helping relationship, the client's capacity to appreciate nuanced humor or paradoxical statements, and the possibilities to repair the relationship should the intervention be misinterpreted.

There are other respectful elements within DBT-WR that practitioners practice and embody. Practitioners commit to not "giving up" on clients. Even though some of the clients who are helped with DBT-WR are challenging to work with and manifest emotions and behaviors related to emotional reactivity, such as anger, despair, idealizing, and dramatically testing boundaries, one "signs up" to facilitate the client's taking a path to live a life worth living. There is full recognition of the demanding nature of this work; thus, the founders of DBT discuss the need for practitioner support and self-care (Comtois et al., 2007; Koerner, 2012; Linehan, 1993) in order to be present and effective.

Similarly, there is recognition that treatment professionals may be emotionally triggered with some clients. Some conflict may emerge on a treatment or service team that is at least partly based on its members having different experiences with a particular client (e.g., one person sees that the client is pleasant and cooperative, another person notes that the client argues with family members). Rather than resorting to polarizing language and setting up camps regarding who is right about a client—"this person is manipulative" versus "no she/he is not"—effort is directed toward radically accepting the views of others, generating *dialogue* to understand different sides of the dialectic, and attempting to "create the appropriate mix of acceptance of the client's vulnerability and change that recognizes the client's strength" (Koerner, 2012, p. 148).

Finally, there is acknowledgment that DBT-WR work also involves case management and clinician support for navigating difficult systemic challenges that clients face (Koerner, 2012). Thus the practitioner becomes an active player in assisting the client's progress with emotion regulation and interpersonal skills, working across the internal and external variables that affect well-being. Advocating and successfully obtaining a service or benefit may contribute mightily to ameliorating concrete factors or social barriers that make emotion regulation that much more difficult. Additionally, the practitioner's engagement in the advocacy process helps build the client's trust in the commitment, the efficacy, and the trustworthiness of the clinician.

Motivational Interviewing

Motivational interviewing is well suited for DBT-WR. The technique incorporates a trans-diagnostic view on client or consumer "readiness to change" (Prochaska, DiClemente, & Norcross, 1992), positing that people progress through various change stages: precontemplation, contemplation, preparation, action, and maintenance (Arkowitz, Westra, Miller, & Rollnick, 2008). Acceptance of the client's process is embedded within motivational interviewing, and client or consumer ambivalence is normalized.

The starting point for motivational interviewing is for the practitioner to drop the agenda of "getting the person to change." Instead of attempting to insert motivation, the practitioner enters a collaborative dialogue with the client and allows motivation to come forward. This less directive stance is preferable because (a) pressure to change can exert a decrease in motivation for change, and (b) many people do not like to be told what to do.

The initial phases of counseling or therapy often correspond to the client's placement in the earlier stages of the change process. In these stages (e.g., precontemplation, contemplation), ambivalence about change is endemic. On the one hand, change may have some appeal because the current state of affairs—the status quo—is painful and challenging, on the other hand the status quo is known and familiar, and change may lead to uncertain and even fear-invoking consequences. Additionally, the person is not sure about whether she or he wants to assume personal ownership of making a change, and may be operating with the frame that change is desired by coercive, nonaccepting others.

In the midst of these dynamics, the practitioner *rolls with client ambivalence* (Arkowitz et al., 2008). We enter a partnership with the client and help sort out the positives and negatives of keeping things the way they are as well as the positives and negatives of changing things. We radically accept that change is hard; that consequences of changing may be challenging; that the person may lack confidence that she or he could actually pull off change (e.g., abstaining from self-harm or substance use); that usually a part of someone, psychologically, is "arguing against" change; and that it is challenging to take ownership of a change effort, especially if one was mandated or pushed into receiving counseling or therapy. Rolling with client ambivalence means that we are comfortable in the murky waters; the client experiences our acceptance and encouragement as well as our fundamental belief in the process.

Motivational interviewing relies heavily on practitioner empathy, nonjudgment, and reflection of the client's reality. It calls on professionals to be comfortable with the present level of client investment toward change as well as the existing level of client ambivalence. Instead of pathologizing a reluctant client as resistant, in denial, or oppositional, we step back from the process and assess the degree to which the nature of the partnership is contributing to the so-called resistance. Motivational interviewing contains the bold assertion that "resistance is relational" (Westra & Dozois, 2008). We ask ourselves if we are pushing too much or going too fast when there appears to be client pushback.

In an environment characterized by curiosity, we may examine how current client behavior is lining up with the individual's values or aspirations. If someone says, "I want to be a better father for my children," we may explore what that looks like for him. This exploration allows him to draw a mental picture and tease out the real possibilities of this occurrence. This kind of work can be more powerful than a practitioner's admonishment about the client's responsibility as a father or the naked assertion of "didn't you say you wanted to be a better father . . . I don't see how hanging out with those folks will help you get there."

We may ask for this client's description of what being a better father would look like, and to discuss how, he imagines, his children would benefit from having him play a positive role in their lives. Additionally, he may imagine what it would feel like to be consistently present in his children's lives, and there would be room to explore his ambivalence about making engaged fatherhood happen. When we discuss a particular behavior with him, we will invite him to reflect and make connections himself (e.g., What about spending time soliciting prostitutes? . . . How much does this relate to your wanting to be a good father or does it feel like this doesn't matter?). When someone's behavior does not line up with aspirations, this process is termed *developing discrepancy*—that is discrepancy between what he asserts that he wishes and his actual behavior. Contrasting behaviors may be explored as to their relationship with hopes and wishes. (I avoid using the word *goals* because it seems to be treatment-driven vocabulary; "Just what *are* your goals, Mr. X?") Again, connecting with the wish to be a better parent: what about attending 12-step meetings regularly? What about asking your child about school . . . ? Ambivalence may return: can I really do this, where is my map to do this, my current behavior is not helpful for my kids but I don't know if I want to or am able to give up my ways. . . .

At this point, we *elicit and explore* the person's own arguments for change as a way to emerge from the ambivalence. Some clients' change talk may be embedded in the conversation such as, "I remember when I did spend time with my daughter—it was nice." Practitioner and client slow down, shine the light on these comments, and ask for elaboration. Sometimes we *elicit* change talk through asking questions, for example, "What was it like when you had a clean period, even one that you may consider extremely short." We may receive a response such as: "I was proud of myself." Within the helping relationship, we slow down, shine the light on *this* particular comment, and ask for elaboration. We may ask a future-oriented question or engage in a visualization, "Imagine life down the road if you were able to stop using" ("cut down on using" in a harm reduction context).

Motivational interviewing is not completely open-ended, and it is not laissez-faire. It leans heavily into the acceptance/ validation part of the acceptance-change dialectic through honoring the client's process and ambivalence. It normalizes that engaging in change is often a dilemma. Motivational interviewing explicitly leans toward change through eliciting and focusing on change talk, as described, and through the *elicit–provide* technique concerning advice. With elicit–provide, practitioners ask clients if it would be okay for the practitioner to give some advice. The act of requesting permission to provide advice is respectful of boundaries and communicates that the advice is provided with the practitioner's intention of being thoughtful and helpful rather than the advice sounding like desperate preaching coming from a reactive and disappointed parent. Arkowitz et al. (2008) state that it is not a question of "if" with elicit–provide but a question of "when and how." Sometimes the delivered advice also contains language of permission. *"Based on what you are telling me about your cravings, some people might suggest that you go to meetings again; maybe you want to consider this."*

While teaching motivational interviewing, some practitioners have raised to me that the style seems too soft and inauthentic and that it seems incongruent vis-à-vis their communication style. Additionally, people have wondered how some communities—particularly communities of color— would respond to a language style that seems "overly therapeutic" or, more directly said, "contrived." At the very least, motivational interviewing points us toward being aware of the potentially negative effects of preaching, confronting, and compromising self-determination. The implications are important when our task as DBT-WR providers is to "teach skills" in order to help people "regulate their emotions." Ultimately, motivational interviewing supports self-efficacy. It communicates that people have wisdom and strengths and that they can find the personal and external resources they need in order engage in life-promoting change.

Substance Abuse Recovery

As noted earlier in the chapter, there are differences regarding recovery philosophy and implementation between the substance abuse and mental health fields. Although SAMHSA (2012) attempted to develop a unified recovery perspective, substance abuse approaches continue to look traditional and not in step with recovery theory on the mental health side. While mental health recovery is characterized by flexibility, client self-determination, and provider–consumer or client relationships that are collaborative, substance abuse intervention emphasizes boundaries, limit setting, and monitoring and compliance. Historically, these substance abuse and mental health arenas operated in independent silos and offered parallel treatment responses for people who were struggling with mental health and substance abuse issues, referred to as dually diagnosed individuals. When individuals must separate parts of themselves—the mental health wellness side and the substance abuse side—into parallel, nonintegrated treatment strands, the prognosis is poor (Burnam & Watkins, 2006; Drake, Mueser, Brunette, & McHugo, 2004). Because of historical practices, cultural differences between substance abuse providers – who are sometimes paraprofessional – and mental health clinicians, varying funding streams and institutional separations, philosophical differences, and differing needs of the populations, it is challenging to provide effective care for people considered dually diagnosed (Conrod & Stewart, 2005).

A view of dual diagnosis prevalence is important to consider. DBT's original population of focus—people diagnosed with borderline personality disorder—had, in one large meta-analysis, a comorbidity rate of 57% for 479 people receiving treatment across diverse settings (Trull, Sher, Minks-Brown, Durbin, & Burr, 2000). Meanwhile, two epidemiological studies report that 61% of people with a bipolar diagnosis qualify for a substance abuse diagnosis. If we start on the substance abuse side, 37% of alcohol abusers and 53% of drug abusers have a serious mental illness (National Alliance on Mental Illness, 2003).

Dual diagnosis work, whether at an agency setting or private practice, often proceeds with a mix of mental health recovery work emphasizing self-determination, client meaning-making, and client–practitioner partnership with substance abuse orientations that stress abstinence, monitoring of usage (perhaps including drug testing), and cognitive work on relapse prevention.

We will highlight various substance abuse recovery issues relevant for DBT-WR application, then briefly discuss how harm reduction practice represents an attempt at implementing more philosophically consonant—across substance abuse and mental health—recovery principles.

Foundations of Substance Abuse Recovery

Substance abuse recovery philosophy largely operates in step with the 12-step movement. Being in recovery means: (a) abstaining from drugs (which includes alcohol), (b) surrendering to the reality of drug addiction, (c) living a spiritually fulfilling life, (d) possessing an internal capacity to be honest, and (e) maintaining integrity in relationships. A person who has ceased using drugs but has made few changes in the other areas is seen as not "being in recovery" (may be labeled as a "dry drunk" in Alcoholics Anonymous language). A person who is making strides in the emotional, interpersonal, and spiritual parts of life but continues some pattern of drug/alcohol use is also characterized as not being in recovery.

A deep exploration of substance abuse work is beyond the scope of this book; however, it is important to look at a few points where DBT-WR may support substance abuse recovery practice and where interesting challenges arise.

Mindfulness practices are beginning to be explored within substance abuse work. Clients may deal with cravings, for example, by noticing them and "developing a spacious, non-judgmental attitude toward all experience . . . (Bowen, Chawla, & Marlatt, 2011, p. 36). Additionally, many relapse experiences occur as a result of emotional triggering states that the individual does not adequately recognize in the moment. For example, a person who becomes bored reacts to this state and begins to fantasize and take steps to find friends and "possibly" use. These kinds of emotional patterns are sometimes subtle and are not captured in traditional cognitive relapse schema that starts with "high-risk stimuli" activating drug-related beliefs (Beck, Wright, Newman, & Liese, 1993).

DBT-WR diligently focuses on the person's developing a capacity for observing, describing, and being with/accepting whatever arises. While grounded in the breath, a person may observe boredom and thoughts about boredom like "I need to relieve this." The person settles into their intention of using Wise Mind and, first, accepts this emotional state and the accompanying thoughts and, second, sees the thought as a thought—one that does not need to be acted upon or dwelled upon. As the process slows down, reactivity diminishes and choices become available. The person allows herself to experience self-compassion for this dilemma, and choose a coping strategy that was part of her safety or relapse plan.

Because substance abuse and mental illness are inseparable for the given person, people who are deeply helped on an emotional level with DBT-WR are helped in their substance abuse recovery. One person who struggled with PTSD and frequently battled with her probation officer learned to regulate her emotions whenever her probation officer (PO) would make critical or noncomplimentary comments. The client had spent a long time working with cognitive strategies that helped her reframe the PO's disposition and that directed her to keep her "eye on the prize"—doing what was necessary to get off probation and maintain her family intact. Various cognitive strategies had minimal utility, as she would become extremely activated with each probation officer interaction as well as despairing and anxious about whether she would be able to move forward or would be held back. In the midst of these periods of emotional distress she would contemplate using again.

DBT-WR made a profound difference for her. She was able to track arising agitation and accept its presence *rather than striving so hard to reason it away.* As distress would arise, her focus became how to apply Wise Mind in order to take care of *herself* in the moment. As a result, she would either initiate actions to improve the moment or engage in bigger picture practices such as, in her case, prayer. Through her implementation of DBT-WR, she was able to defuse from the story that often dominated the day and hijacked her emotional well-being. The focus on taking care of herself and regulating her emotions was more effective than pursuing cognitive strategies that kept her in the highly stressful loop of reasoning the degree to which her fears were realistic, and so on.

Being less "stressed out" overall meant that she fantasized less about relapsing and was able to maintain focus and direction regarding personal recovery and wellness. Staying true to the recovery principle of respecting and honoring client wisdom, she and another client ended up presenting some DBT-WR concepts to staff in an intra-agency training.

DBT–WR and Substance Abuse Treatment Dialectics

There are some interesting comparisons related to the dialectical dynamics between DBT-WR and traditional substance abuse perspectives. Both views emphasize acceptance. Within the 12-step tradition, one is to accept "powerlessness over drugs and alcohol" and accepts and surrenders to the reality that something beyond the person's own self is needed to heal. Finally, one learns acceptance of self after, in the fourth step, revealing shortcomings and character flaws in, most often, a written statement. Acceptance of self is enhanced when the recovering addict realizes that neither the person they read their statement to nor their higher power will abandon them. Of course, radical acceptance is integral in DBT-WR as well. Emotions and thoughts arise, and we see them for what they are—in a sense we surrender to them, to use 12-step language. We experience the validation of the practitioner who appreciates the client's internal life. In DBT-WR, we emphasize self-compassion for whatever arises in our minds, which we do not ultimately have control or "power" over.

The formal or informal cognitive tradition embedded within the 12 steps, however, offers some differences. One internalizes the label of alcoholic or drug addict, and the medicine for this disease is to stay away from "people, places, and things" that put one at risk. Some of these "things" are thoughts and emotions that may be fertile ground for using or relapsing. Thus, some people adopt the strategy of walling off "stinking thinking" or boredom or sadness. Think positively, call your sponsor, pray, go to a meeting, let go of the "fuck-its," focus on today, let go and let God. The gray area is experienced as dangerous because, according to the 12-step approach, the addictive mind that finds itself in this kind of space will gather steam and make a push to use.

Thus, a few people struggling with addiction may be ambivalent about DBT-WR because it seems challenging to integrate mindfulness of emerging personal processes with instructions to keep it simple and focus on turning their life over to their higher power. There are possibilities to integrate this dialectic. Mindfulness of arising internal phenomena helps one emotionally settle, and actually opens up possibilities to connect with one's higher power. Although apparently opening the field for different thoughts, emotions, and behaviors, Wise Mind and mindfulness makes it *less* likely that someone will become hijacked by their emotions and respond reactively. Nearly everyone struggling with substance abuse comes away with this view—that DBT-WR skills are quite helpful, not only for their day-to-day wellness but also for relapse prevention.

A program more limited in scope and time frame (eight sessions), mindfulness-based relapse prevention (MBRP) showed some promising results in the areas mentioned. In a randomized study, MBRP was compared to a traditional aftercare program offered at a particular site. The *reduction* in craving for the MBRP participants was significantly greater than for the participants in the standard after-care program through the 4-month follow-up period. MBRP people also reported that they acted with less reactivity and were more aware and accepting than the standard aftercare counterparts. MBRP members also used alcohol and drugs significantly less through the 4-month follow-up period; however, usage rate differences disappeared at the 4-month mark (Bowen et al., 2011). In order to sustain positive results, this study perhaps points to the need for extending the time frame of the work (such as 15 sessions for DBT-WR), for making the application more extensive (DBT-WR's ongoing integration with treatment and having a broader scope than MBRP's aftercare focus), and for connecting to supportive structures beyond formal treatment.

Substance abuse and mental health recovery differentially approach the dialectic of structured guidelines versus mutual discovery and client–practitioner partnership. As previously mentioned, substance abuse recovery, even in the SAMHSA (2012) definition, involves setting the standard of client abstinence. A client in this treatment environment, though motivational interviewing techniques may be utilized, still is expected to *behaviorally conform* to abstinence markers. Positive drug/alcohol tests are somewhat tolerated in the early stages of treatment; however, a significant period of clean time and consistent attendance at 12-step programs or similar events is eventually expected and is necessary in order to "graduate." The client's version of reality—that taking a couple of drinks is less damaging and dangerous than doing methamphetamine on the street—is not validated and is, in fact, discounted. Abstinence-based work is an either-or proposition. Even if there were a philosophical concession that a couple of drinks were less damaging (at least it is not illegal), the theory is that when the addict crosses the line, there is no such thing as responsible and contained use. The client's exploration of the drinking alternative is labeled as bargaining, seen as indicative of a lack of commitment to maintain sobriety, portrayed as denial of the nature of the problem, and questioned as a back-door path to start using at the same level again.

Therefore, the clients' job is to surrender—surrender to powerlessness, surrender to the notion of being an addict, and surrender to the structure of the treatment program. If clients do not surrender, they are viewed as pursuing their own agendas, which involve small-minded scheming and irresponsible fulfillment of desires.

Abstinence oriented approaches have helped hundreds of thousands of people. Some people likely cannot function in the vague environment of controlled or responsible substance use. Many claim that without the rituals, rules, and structures of programs, the courts, testing, and 12 steps, they would default to the rules of the addict mind, which asserts "I want it now" or default to the rules of the streets. Sometimes the container of the program will determine the degree of structure that is expected regarding substance use, and sometimes there is latitude. In individual work, it may become apparent that harm reduction attempts do not yield the benefits that clients were hoping for (e.g., more stable relationships, fewer health or legal crises, enhanced capacity to function with a clear mind during the day, a sense that life was improving). *DBT has combined with traditional 12-step work and has achieved promising results*, particularly in treatment retention (over simple DBT groups for substance users) and in emotion regulation and reduction in self-harm behaviors (over traditional 12-step groups) (McMain, Sayrs, Dimeff, & Linehan, 2007).

Harm Reduction   In general, however, "DBT does not require that (people) contract to stop all drug use . . ." (Dimeff & Koerner, 2007, p. 167). Harm reduction approaches may be integrated with DBT, and DBT per se does not describe substance use as a disease nor insist on people calling themselves "addicts." (Dimeff & Koerner, 2007). The harm-reduction approach is consonant with the mental health recovery perspective in that it is client-centered and more reliant on the client–practitioner partnership and mutual discovery than on structure and consequences.

The emphasis on acceptance and validation appears to be the major point of convergence between harm reduction and DBT-WR. Drug use, for example, may be mutually framed as an adaptive, understandable strategy for emotion regulation and the amelioration of stress (Denning & Little, 2012). Combined with motivational interviewing, client-practitioner engagement occurs to explore the pros and cons of various levels of substance use. In an environment of radical acceptance, the client may be willing to consider the possibility that "regulating use" is not, nor has it been, a viable strategy. Some may choose abstinence because of their honest realization that this is the only way to live a life that is workable. In a harm reduction approach, the practitioner stays "one step behind" the client; thus, it is the client who makes this determination (Denning & Little, 2012).

Many case managers, service coordinators, clinical social workers, counselors, psychologists and psychiatrists of community mental health programs work within a harm reduction context (see Denning & Little, 2012, for an authoritative treatment of harm reduction practice). As they apply DBT-WR in these settings, they blend harm reduction philosophy—emphasizing active use of self, high tolerance of clients' being who they are and doing what they do, maximizing client participation and self-determination—with the structure of DBT-WR activities and lessons. In DBT-WR group settings, maximum flexibility may not be possible in order for the group to have integrity. Thus, clients or consumers affiliated with these settings will make the empowered choice regarding whether they wish to participate given the group's structure.

In general the DBT-WR practitioner needs to embrace the dialectic between structure and responsiveness. A structure that is predictable, has some rhythm (e.g., beginning, middle, and end of group), and prepared activities and basic rules may be a responsive way for meeting needs. However, an emphasis on responsiveness may lead to modifications in structure, thus becoming a structure in motion. Embracing the dialectical relationship of DBT-WR structure with clinician responsiveness to individual client recovery is captured in the metaphor about how the strings of a guitar need to be adjusted in order to make beautiful music. Too much flexibility, or too loose, and you cannot make beautiful music; too much structure, or too tight, and the strings break.

CHAPTER Four
Accounting for Trauma

Overview

Across mental health practices, potential beneficiaries of DBT-WR struggle with the effects of trauma. Throughout these settings, women more frequently have been victimized by traumatic events. For those engaged in substance abuse, for example, women are three times more likely than men to have a posttraumatic stress disorder (PTSD) diagnosis. Women who are using drugs and alcohol commonly find themselves in a "downward spiral . . . their substance use may increase vulnerability to new traumas, which in turn can lead to more substance use" (Najavits, 2002, p. 2). Most women who are dually diagnosed with PTSD and substance abuse have experienced childhood physical and/ or sexual abuse while most dually diagnosed men have been victims of violence or war trauma (Briere & Scott, 2006).

Trauma often plays a role in the development of borderline personality disorder (BPD) as well (van der Kolk, MacFarlane, & Weisaeth, 1996) and BPD's emergence has been conceptualized as resting on a childhood foundation of trauma and chronic terror (Herman, Perry, & Van der Kolk, 1989).

Zanarini et al. (1997) stated that 91% of people with the BPD diagnosis reported childhood abuse.

It is important to mention, however, that an identifiable trauma background is not required for a BPD diagnosis (Briere & Scott, 2006) and childhood trauma is not a necessary contributor to BPD for an individual who already had biological vulnerability regarding emotion regulation (Dimeff & Koerner, 2007). Regardless of whether *childhood* trauma occurred, adults with serious mental illness are at increased risk of victimization and trauma (Sells, Rowe, Fisk, & Davidson, 2003).

There are various reasons to specifically account for trauma within dialectical behavior therapy for wellness and recovery (DBT-WR). First, when clients understand how trauma impacts emotion regulation challenges, their own experiences with emotional lability are normalized. Second, basic neuroscience explanations regarding trauma invite people into the thought process behind DBT-WR as well as the emotion regulation endeavor. Clients appreciate and feel empowered that they are involved in "rewiring" their brain. Third, the bare mention of trauma contributes to the client validation portion of the DBT-WR validation–change dialectic. Especially in DBT-WR groups, where the practitioner does not intimately know the client's or consumer's story, just acknowledging the reality that trauma is likely part of the lives of many people in the room speaks to the intensely lived experience of individual group members. Fourth, keeping trauma in mind helps practitioners tune in to the degree to which emotion regulation may be practiced in the here-and-now, and that events occurring during group or individual sessions may be triggering. Fifth, principles of grounding or pendulation are important to implement within DBT-WR sessions. Keeping in mind the client's "resilient zone" (Miller-Karas & Leitch, 2009) may help practitioners with here-and-now regulation efforts and may inform responsive strategies for helping to stabilize or settle down a person so that she or he may benefit from DBT-WR.

Before we address these points, it is important to grapple with definitions. The brain refers to a specific physical entity, as well as its circuitry, and activity. While the mind is "considered as a *subjectively perceived* functional entity, based ultimately on physical processes . . . it governs the total organism and its interaction with the environment" (Siegel, 2003, p. 8, italics mine).

The notion of mind transcends physical brain processes and activity and involves the way that spirit, intellect, and sense of self interact with the world. The "subjectively perceived" part of the definition depicts why we say "mindfulness." The mind can be subjectively perceived whereas similar perception of one's brain is not possible.

Trauma to Normalize Emotion Regulation Challenges

Clients are often struggling with their emotional lives and the behaviors and consequences that flow from them. Others have labeled them and they have labeled themselves as *troubled* in one way or another, and their reactive and not well regulated emotional states reinforce the degree to which life and their wellness seem to constantly turn on a moment's notice. Trauma provides an explanatory framework for many clients about how they have arrived at the point at which they find themselves.

Ironically, information about trauma lays the groundwork for "a focus on potential rather than pathology" (Najavits, 2002, p. 12). People learn that they have overcome a lot in their lives and that they have been heroic to accomplish what they have. They also learn that some of their emotional responses are *understandable* given what they have endured. Fight–freeze–flight responses are kinds of adaptations that have helped them survive difficult circumstances. Even people who have not had *Diagnostic and Statistical Manual of Mental Disorders* (DSM)–eligible PTSD precursor experiences find value in this discussion. Struggling with mental health challenges, feeling stigmatized and isolated, moving in and out of despair and feelings of chronic emptiness, being part of a group that is denigrated and collectively traumatized in society (e.g., Brave Heart, 2007; Ina, 1999), experiencing dislocations and frightening uncertainty, and struggling through frequent bouts of anger provide a connection point with people who formally meet PTSD criteria.

When clients and consumers operate from a base of appreciation regarding who they are, where they came from, and how much they have persevered, they are prepared to cultivate greater self-compassion. There are contributing reasons that may explain how mental wellness has been compromised; those reasons can be externalized—that is to say, not seen as part of their "failed, pathetic selves"—and new responses may be learned and practiced. "Oh, so *that* is why I act that way," one client said as she connected screaming at her boyfriend the previous evening for buying her a fish taco ("he should know I don't like fish") with the day's DBT-WR lesson on trauma and emotional reactivity.

Although a basic understanding of trauma and emotional reactivity is covered in DBT-WR, the intended effect is not to demoralize clients (see Najavits, 2002). The emphasis is on developing compassion for one's self, gaining a sense of universality with others who have similarly suffered, and internalizing the optimistic message that emotional life and skillful response is achievable.

Neuroscience Engenders Hope and Interest

A surprising qualitative outcome regarding DBT-WR groups was clients' mentioning the degree to which they appreciated being shown a model of the brain. The discussion accompanying the figure of the brain (see Lesson 1 in Chapter 6) highlighted that the amygdala may be overactive for some people who have struggled through trauma, and that enhanced amygdala activity meant a neurochemical response that produced more stress. The task of DBT-WR was to change the way our brain worked. DBT-WR would help mobilize our prefrontal cortex in order to help us (a) experience enhanced mood and sense of well-being, (b) boost motivation, (c) improve judgment, (d) increase overall calmness, and (e) provide greater brain integration with the amygdala. Not only did this description prove helpful and motivating, but clients believed that the inclusion of this material for discussion demonstrated the practitioner's respect for their intelligence (Richards & Sehr, 2011).

Wise Mind, in essence, is described as "hanging out more in the prefrontal cortex." The primary vehicle for making this happen is the cultivation of mindfulness. We are to become, as Daniel Siegel (2010) says, *friends with our minds* through being able to observe arising thoughts and emotions, and to accept them, face them, and effectively deal with them.

Although nothing can be done to change past experiences of victimization and trauma, we are empowered to engage in the miracle of rewiring our brains. The notion of neuroplasticity suggests a path of hope and possibility for people who once believed that their patterns of emotional responses were an unchangeable reality.

Being able to gather the mind and observe one's process in the moment means less vulnerability to becoming hijacked by the mind and engaging in reactive, unskillful action. We learn that through staying in the moment—a parallel lesson to the 12-step mantra of "one day at a time"—our situation is more workable, balanced, and calm.

In essence, the ability to observe the mind as well as create new pathways enhances the system's complexity. Perpetual overstimulation that occurs in chaotic or traumatic environments stresses the brain as does monotony or sameness. People tend to experience anxiety in chaotic environments as well as in boring or monotonous ones. **Complexity** ideally "flows between boredom and anxiety" (Siegel, 2003, p. 5) so as to reduce stress and create new neuron firing patterns. Clients thus learn to soothe when highly activated or overwhelmed and to "plug in" and find resources when understimulated or depressed.

The Special Case of Boredom

When I take the pulse of the group through observation and during a group summation period, I am assessing for boredom and anxiety. Boredom is sometimes subtle and leads to flight (mentally checking out), freeze (dissociated gaze), or fight (acting out, restless). It is important to tune into client statements or indications of boredom, without practitioner defensiveness. For many, boredom is a major trigger to use substances or to contemplate self-harm. Offering opportunities for complexity may include the practitioner encouraging the client to engage in the following six practices:

1. Mindful observation and acceptance of boredom; in other words, nothing needs to be done—notice how boredom arises and recedes.

2. Finding ways to plug back in; maybe boredom means you are not paying attention to the reality that there are beautiful beings in the room engaged in the remarkable endeavor of trying to understand their lives and make their lives better.

3. Examining intention—how much do you want to show up and live in your Wise Mind?

4. Skillfully fashioning a suggestion (the client is to do this) that may contribute to a new direction for the group (but being prepared to let go of the outcome—that is, let go of *insisting* that the group moves in a direction that you desire).

5. Soothing yourself in the midst of the boredom. Notice the stories that may arise (e.g., this group sucks, I am tired of this crap because it is pointless, who is this doofus leading the

group?) and see if you can let them go rather than investing further in them.

6. Notice if watching the clock is the most effective way to deal with boredom.

These suggestions and inquiries are provocative efforts at changing the way people may respond to "being bored" rather than maintaining conditions that contribute to clients' habitually defaulting or falling into their "well-worn groove." Although well worn, being stuck in these grooves or habitual patterns may be stressful and unenjoyable.

Acknowledgment of Trauma and Extreme Stress Validates Clients

The validation/acceptance and change dialectic is important to emphasize throughout DBT-WR work. In skills-based "training" or curriculums, the implicit core message may be that the client or consumer is in need of fixing because of inherent deficits, or, in this case, "emotion regulation challenges." Although the DBT-WR presented here acknowledges strengths, personal coping strategies, and a recovery-oriented view, the curriculum-oriented nature of the work may crowd out part of the client's intense personal narrative coming into the room in favor of material regarding present moment mindfulness and coping—in other words, the *change* part of the dialectic. Acknowledging trauma and its potential impact *validates* the struggles that many people have dealt with and have, to some degree, overcome.

Trauma survivors have experienced the unspeakable. Not only does the survivor encounter the societal message that people do not want to hear or be witness to the person's story, but the *perpetrator's* outright denial of traumatic events, in the case of human-inflicted abuse, is an integral part of the individual's victimization (Mollica, 2006). Very few individuals, when confronted with the harm that they have perpetrated upon another, come forward with, "Yes, I did this, and I am very sorry." Instead, not only does the trauma victim deal with the consequences of feeling under threat and experiencing that there is little reliable "ground" to stand on, but she tolerates the additional humiliation, from the very person who has victimized her, who in effect says, "You are making this up . . . you are exaggerating things . . . *you* are creating the problems with all your complaining . . . you need to stop blaming people for all your issues."

Dynamics related to invalidation may build on internal shame and humiliation that appears to be integral regardless of the trauma suffered. People who are victimized by natural disasters, accidents, or sudden acute states of illness seem to experience shame for merely having the experience and for feeling vulnerable. In a state of disequilibrium and fear, it seems more likely that one suffers humiliation and shame when reaching out rather than feeling calmness and confidence. According to Mollica (2006), dynamics connecting *shame* with *trauma* (including trauma without human perpetrators) seem so universal that a biological and perhaps evolutionary contribution needs to be considered to account for the cross-cultural shame–trauma connection. In some instances language regarding "dependency" and cultural norms about the "selfishness" implied in asking for help (rather than being stoic) accentuate survivor shame and embarrassment.

The acknowledgment and exploration of trauma's effects with a concurrent DBT-WR focus on skill-building and present-oriented involvement offers a middle path for clients straddling between what Herman (1997) refers to as the simultaneous inclination to "tell all" and to say nothing. In other words, we give voice to the reality of trauma through mentioning its presence and through discussing and normalizing the degree to which trauma contributes to emotion regulation challenges. To the degree that there is a connection between trauma and emotion regulation struggles, clients understand the potential source of their challenges and develop compassion for themselves as they grapple with present-focused DBT-WR lessons and possibilities. In this manner, trauma comes into the room. Its contribution is acknowledged, and the work ahead to deal with its effects is articulated through the curriculum. Depending on the therapeutic or helping context, the particular trauma story may be more fully explored and processed in a designated time (and perhaps with another practitioner) beyond the DBT-WR curriculum.

Being Mindful of Trauma in the Here-and-Now

Accounting for trauma in the here-and-now involves the practitioner's awareness of client activation in the room. Aggressive fellow clients, comments from mental health practitioners perceived as challenging or judgmental, insensitive or threatening treatment structures, raised voices, emotion-invoking material, and confrontational questions may provoke a strong reaction from a client who is on high alert for danger. The practitioner's assessment, nondefensiveness, and skillful navigation of behavior that is possibly trauma based are important.

Your intention, as a practitioner, may be sincerely directed toward creating safety and not activating a particular client; however, your observations or the client's direct responses indicate that your involvement or the way you are conducting the group or individual session sets conditions in motion for client reactivity. Sometimes we learn about this process through a client's angry comments or direct violation of rules or norms (fight), or a client's disengagement, laissez-faire approach, or desire to be invisible (freeze or flight). Our job is to radically accept what is occurring and what we are observing. We attempt to be open to what is happening without reacting with our own fight–freeze–flight responses, such as (a) immediately intervening to make something happen and change things;

(b) denying that anything important is happening; or (c) fantasizing about how good the group would be if the "offending" person were not in it. If we notice such thoughts and inclinations arising, we let them go and return to our intention of being skillfully responsive with our clients. We may have to let go of our defensiveness if we have been criticized, or our sense of inadequacy if the client does not seem to be gaining from the DBT-WR experience.

We then practice from the dialectic of acceptance and change regarding our client. There is a degree to which we want to let the client feel that she can show up as she is. She does not have to be a "good client"—that is, passively conform to practitioner or agency demands and expectations—and does not have to be maximally engaged each moment. On some level we know that just validating her and the way she shows up to the individual or group session has value. However, *if the treatment experience provides an opportunity for the client to practice the kind of reactivity, avoidance, or dysregulation that she or he practices in the outside world, the treatment context may have limited usefulness.* As practitioners, we begin to understand that engaging with the topic of emotional reactivity means that we sometimes move into the reactivity that is occurring in the room. Talking about reactivity as if it is always about something "out there" means that we can miss important learning opportunities.

Therefore, as practitioners and clients, *we work together* to establish a safe environment that encourages involvement. We are quite careful not to be intrusive to the point where practitioner actions are interpreted as being critical. We also consider that because of cultural influences and differences in verbal confidence and anxiety levels, client engagement may tilt more in the direction of mindful listening than toward active verbal participation. The therapeutic environment *celebrates* how the person shows up, offers opportunities to address the environment to make it feel safe, *and* offers *challenges* that are not too stressful in order for people to practice skillful engagement in the change process. This kind of treatment approach is congruent with the acceptance/validation and change dialectic encouraged throughout DBT-WR.

Resilient Zone

DBT-WR is not a trauma-focused therapy; however, many people in DBT-WR contexts have been victimized by trauma; thus, principles of deactivation are relevant. If clients experience an *overall sense of well-being* while they are in DBT-WR, they may be more likely to internalize emotion regulation lessons and to carry these lessons out into their lives.

Miller-Karas & Leitch (2009) developed the concept of the "resilient zone within which our thoughts, feelings and sensations are working well together" (p. 28). When people are "bumped out" of the resilient zone, they may be stuck on either *high arousal* (hyperactivity, hypervigilance, rage, and panic) or *low arousal* (depression, disconnection, fatigue, numbness). There are different methods that help people "find" the resilient zone, including grounding and pendulation.

Grounding helps someone who is in either high or low arousal. The process helps the person occupy her or his own body and connect with the support that is inherent in the environment—the ground. Grounding serves to help a client who, during a session, is highly distressed and agitated, or who is reliving a traumatic experience and is becoming overwhelmed. Usually, the practitioner leads the client through the process of noticing points of contact with the body (e.g., the buttocks on the chair and the feet on the ground) as well as noticing the breath slowing down. The practitioner's voice slows and refers to the way that the ground and chair offer support in order for the person to settle and begin to relax. At that point the practitioner may lead the client(s) to bring attention to parts of their body that feel comfortable or at least neutral (Miller-Karas & Leitch, 2009).

One central element of grounding is the temporary respite from stimulating and provocative content. Clients who generalize this process and apply it *outside* the counseling context realize that they may, in their day-to-day lives, seek sanctuary from emotionally triggering events and not "spin out" to high levels of despair or rage. At times and with some individuals, radically accepting emotions, thoughts, and processes is too subtle in the midst of a crisis or stress hormone–charged situation. Grounding offers an embodied *respite* from pain (e.g., notice the beautiful sky around you) that may be more effective than *being with* experience and mindfully connecting to breath.

Just as with mindfulness exercises, grounding exercises are introduced with the encouragement that there is no evaluation or grade that will be given regarding "how well" clients ground themselves. People are encouraged to notice that these kinds of performance-oriented thoughts may arise, and to let them go.

Pendulation is another useful concept offered within the Trauma Resilience Model (TRM) and refers to the need for balancing highly charged and activating material with more neutral and safe content. In the case of directly processing trauma (not typically done in DBT-WR), pendulation allows the person to regroup, not get overwhelmed, and effectively deal with trauma material—manageable bits at a time.

For DBT-WR, pendulation orients the practitioner to "swing back" from periods of in-session intensity to a session environment that feels safe and not so emotionally stimulating. (See Miller-Karas & Leitch, 2009, regarding these issues and the vast range of TRM applications—from private-practice contexts to field work with Haitian earthquake survivors).

Pendulation has practical application for DBT-WR that goes beyond processing someone's traumatic memories. In one particular group where people were reviewing their interpersonal approaches, some clients realized the degree to which they practiced interpersonal behaviors that the clients themselves could see were insensitive, noncaring, nonempathic, and abusive. In the middle of the group's exploration of their various behaviors, two different clients indicated that this work had been extremely difficult and stressful and that a few times they had just wanted to tune out. However, they answered the questions sincerely and indicated positive ways in which they could not only enhance their awareness in various interpersonal situations, but could also be more responsive to others. After a period of serious exploration, they asked, "Could we just move off this exercise for a while?"

There were two possible responses that seemed viable. First, I could ask the clients to sit with the intensity and the stress so that they could develop confidence to face it and hold it. This response type is supported by a traditional substance abuse treatment mentality that says "growth is going to be hard work; toughen up and do what it takes. Maybe getting 'ripped up' inside about how you have been treating people poorly is a *good* thing."

The second response type elevated the importance of the clients' stated needs and would take into account the degree to which the material and group environment was stressing them. I chose this response because (a) I considered it positive and insightful that the clients could tune into their own stress level and that they had, in fact, utilized mindfulness skills; (b) they fashioned a reasonable request—that is, they used the very interpersonal skills we had been speaking about rather than act out or derail the process; and (c) I considered that pendulation had relevance here. The emotional intensity was high and people were becoming dysregulated. Rather than move solidly out of the clients' resilient zone, it made sense to respond to their request and "take the foot off the gas."

Pendulation, then, is about moving from high activation to lower activation. (It may also refer to moving into more intense engagement for an individual or group that is disengaged or exhibiting low energy.) Through talking about the process rather than the content of the lesson, through validating the clients' sincere work on the exercise, through taking a few deep breaths, and through ceding to their wishes to move on, the activation level within the group lessened. During the group's summary at the close of the group, some serious reflection reemerged. Interpersonal skills lessons clearly had been digested.

In retrospect, this approach had additional ramifications. It honored the clients' point of view and their personal articulations regarding what would lead to present-moment wellness. Their willingness to do the difficult work, monitor their own emotional state, make a responsible request, and benefit from enhanced, in-the-moment emotion regulation was a valuable process.

Seen within a *recovery paradigm*, this chosen direction turns responsibility for the client's progress over to the clients themselves. Partnership and collaboration are valued over practitioner-led agenda setting and session management. Stepping away from the curriculum not only provided an experience of being cared for; it also opened up possibilities for the healing benefits of laughter—the ultimate pendulation activity.

Richard Mollica (2006) discusses the importance of humor from his worldwide experience working with traumatized populations in places such as Cambodia and Bosnia:

> As demonstrated by extensive research, laughter and humor are therapeutic. While this reality has found its way into cancer wards and into the treatment of other serious medical disorders, it has barely entered the doorway of modern psychiatry. Mental health practitioners are likely afraid that humor will be seen as insensitive to an already vulnerable person. Yet without humor and the joy it triggers, an additional aid to recovery is lost. . . . The true place of laughter in recovery is a simple exercise like the daily walk [and is an] aid in the healing of physical and mental disorders. (pp. 205–206)

Teaching radical acceptance and mindfulness skills, skillfully balancing the dialectic between validation and change, effectively dealing with boundaries, experiencing emotions regarding practitioner ineffectiveness, and establishing a safe container for people who are in despair or rage requires a deliberate and thoughtful use-of-self. The next chapter discusses use-of-self themes relevant for DBT-WR.

Five

Clinician's Use-of-Self: Foundation for Effective Practice

Let the mind be the mind.
Behind its restless activity,
just one layer deeper
is stillness, and beneath
even that, is an ocean
of mystery and truth.

Danna Faulds
(Reprinted with permission; may be photo-
copied as part of practitioner's lessons.)

Clients develop an in-depth understanding about dialectical behavior therapy for wellness and recovery (DBT-WR) through watching their therapist or counselor. It is, therefore, important for practitioners to be congruent with the principles we, as practitioners, espouse, such as being radically accepting in the midst of arising difficulties. An authentic, accepting, and caring self may be the most powerful tool that mental health practitioners may have (Bertolino & Miller, 2012; Duncan, Miller, & Sparks, 2004;); this chapter will discuss how to cultivate and integrate an effective use-of-self in the DBT-WR context.

DBT suggests ways of being for mental health practitioners *ourselves*. Upon making this realization, clinicians decide to dedicate more effort to self-reflection, personal mindfulness practices, and ways in which to incorporate radical acceptance into our own lives. We also come to realize that how we carry ourselves in moment-to-moment practice with clients has an enormous impact. I have had many practitioners tell me during trainings that they never really understood DBT until they encountered some of the use-of-self lessons that we will cover here.

Strong Back, Soft Front

Strong back, soft front is a concept developed by Joan Halifax, PhD, through her many years of work as a practitioner, theoretician, and trainer within the hospice field as well as through her involvement in prisons. Strong back and soft front has special utility for DBT-WR because it parallels the dialectical dynamic of acceptance and change. Many human service practitioners find this language memorable and immensely practical (see Bein, 2008).

Strong back helps us deal with the uncertainty embedded in mental health practice or therapy. From moment to moment we do not know what we will face, the effects of our involvement, or the cognitive and emotional processes unfolding within our client(s). Strong back allows us to solidly take our seat in the middle of this uncertainty. We can imagine ourselves, sitting with a settled mind and an erect, not rigid, posture. We may even notice our own trepidation, insecurity, and confusion about how to proceed; however, with our strong back we have trust in the process and in the here-and-now.

Ultimately, our strong back is a container for our own doubts and the doubts and emotional turmoil of the other. With our own capacity to maintain calmness and balance, we, with some confidence, meet the moment and whatever the moment offers.

Dr. Martin Luther King expressed the strong back sentiment through an account of his leadership during the bus boycott of the 1960s. In the midst of threats on his life,

violence against the African American community, growing impatience because of the limited initial results of the
boycott, and a lack of clarity about how to proceed, Dr. King
prepared to address a large African American crowd in a
Montgomery, Alabama, church. Dr. King on that day drew
from his mentor's advice regarding the foundation principle for delivering a meaningful sermon: "Open your mouth
and God will speak for you" (Carson, 1998, p. 61). Dr. King
arrived that night with no notes in his hand; he trusted
his strong back and that if he brought himself fully to the
moment, the needed words would be revealed. He later
reflected on the evening's events and stated "this speech had
evoked more response than any speech or sermon I had ever
delivered" (Carson, 1998, p. 61).

"Open your mouth and God will speak for you" may be
literally integrated and appreciated by some. Others may see
it metaphorically or would prefer other language. From a Zen
perspective the meaning is:

> Trust that if you bring yourself with a strong back to the
> present moment, you will tap into the universe's reser-
> voir of wisdom and skillful means. (Bein, 2008, p. 13)

Strong back has profound implications for modeling emotion regulation for our clients and consumers. Life continually
unfolds in uncertain and unpredictable ways. We cannot even
fully control thoughts and emotional states that arise within
us. What we *can* do is develop confidence that we can skillfully meet and respond to whatever arises without going too
far astray (i.e., becoming too reactive). We continue to take our
seat and face our lives, preferring the truth of what is unfolding in front of us to denial or other means of escape.

Strong back is the mountain ground. We embody the solidity of the mountain, yet, just as the mountain changes through
mud slides and animal and plant life cycles, we dynamically
change. We transcend our fight-or-flight tendencies and sink

into our calm breath and, like the mountain, stay put. We listen to the client's struggles and aspirations; we are aware of our own doubts arising; and we sincerely proceed with a still, settled mind in the midst of uncertainty.

The structure, protocol, and boundaries germane to the client–practitioner encounter are strong back elements. The rules about what clients and practitioners can and cannot do as well as the reason for our meeting provides definition and purpose to our coming together. Yes, we are to cultivate a positive, meaningful, and caring relationship, but we are also there to get some work done. The demand for work (Shulman, 1999) inherent in the helping relationship is strong back. These elements are similar to the *change* part of the validation–change dialectic. There are times when we ultimately hold ourselves and our clients accountable; that is our strong back being expressed.

Ironically, practitioners appreciate their strong back as a resource in the midst of their own fear or trepidation regarding mental health practice situations. Embodying a strong back, one enters a situation, fears and all, sensing internally that it is acceptable to have hesitance or doubt. In the midst of feeling unconfident, strong back helps us persevere.

Our strong back is needed to allow our soft front or open heart to flourish. Practitioners early in their career sometimes lead with soft front, but their boundaries may not be well developed so they can feel taken advantage of or be unclear about their roles. Conversely, highly experienced practitioners who have suffered disappointment and frustration may lean too heavily in the direction of strong back and, in doing so, stifle their open-hearted soft front.

> Our soft front allows us to be truly touched by our clients' lives. We begin to actually experience our clients' pain because as we sit—open hearted—with our clients we deeply realize that their pain is ultimately the world's pain. (Bein, 2008, p. 16)

This soft front allows us to universalize people's struggles and triumphs and to see into the depths of people and their aspirations, well beyond the diagnostic or deviant labels that have followed them for years.

Our soft front is about love and optimism. We solidly bring ourselves to the moment (strong back) and open our hearts to make a connection and genuinely care. Soft front provides the practitioner's heart and positive disposition contributing to the client's felt experience of validation and acceptance. Our soft front projects that the world is better off for the existence of the particular client and carries our hopes that the client experiences a life worth living. Making contact with the practitioner's soft front helps build client acceptance and compassion for self, often in spite of a history of invalidation and victimization.

Our capacity to be aware of and balance our strong back and soft front is parallel to our skill of balancing our emphasis on change and service structure integrity, on the one hand, with client acceptance and spontaneous responsiveness, on the other.

Finally, the practitioner's manifestation of strong back and soft front provides an emotion regulation model for clients. Maintaining our emotional and mental stability in the midst of turmoil (strong back) while maintaining a willingness to engage and projecting a sense of possibilities (soft front) embody qualities of resilience and emotional regulation. We hold the intention of maintaining our strong back and soft front in order to effectively use our professional self in the DBT-WR context.

Use-of-Self Interface With Radical Acceptance

Acceptance provides the ground for change within DBT-WR. On the deepest personal level, people are inclined to respond skillfully when we are settled in our own personal process—that is, we essentially feel accepting about who we are. From this spot of overall personal acceptance, we respond flexibly and skillfully to arising situations, not because we are fundamentally deficient or inadequate, but because we deserve to build "a life worth living."

These principles ultimately pertain to DBT-WR clients and consumers as well as mental health providers. If practitioners are basing their self-esteem on client outcomes, if they act defensively in the face of threats to the ego, or if they are relying on client praise for obtaining a sense of wellness, then they are going to struggle establishing a container of acceptance. Practitioners gain comfort accepting others because we have gained comfort with ourselves. Even in the midst of client expressions of frustrations, complaints, acting-out episodes, and varying levels of "noncompliance," mental health practitioners and therapists communicate the message that the client is fundamentally accepted and appreciated.

Practitioners maintain emotional stability and steadfast radical acceptance of clients through nonreactive acceptance of one's personal arising thoughts and emotions. In other words, we teach nonreactivity through being nonreactive ourselves (as practitioners). We maintain the discipline of attending to and facing emotions and thoughts and then of consciously adopting strategies to address them. We seek to maintain a degree of resilience so that situations with clients or client groups do not lead to practitioner reactivity.

However, some client behavior manages to affect us deeply and knock us off center. Particular clients or consumers struggling with emotional regulation do a good job at helping us (practitioners) experience their internal world. As clients convert their agitation about their lives or the DBT-WR process into complaints, arguments, or efforts at derailment, practitioners may become agitated. Agitation is not a problem; we have the opportunity to continue moving forward through accepting personal agitation and responding skillfully. When we succeed in containing both our client's and our own agitation, we create powerful lessons regarding emotion regulation possibilities.

Clients often expect different results when they are expressing agitation or acting out. For some, these kinds of behaviors are precursors to power struggles where each side ups the ante and emotional or physical violence may ensue. Others have had the experience that agitation or expression of frustration leads to increased punitive treatment, which, in turn, leads to increased frustration, despair, and possible emotional meltdown. Skillful emotional regulation on the practitioner's part may create a surprising result as well as a here-and-now experience of the benefits of emotion regulation and skillful response.

Containment and successful resolution of difficulty contributes to a group environment that is "welcoming the whole person" (Malekoff, 2004, p. 39), and lets members see that acceptance and moving toward emotion regulation are the norms. Teens, particularly those referred to groups, are accustomed to violating norms and receiving reactive and punitive responses. One DBT-WR teen participant commented, after the group terminated, on how I had accepted him even after he exclaimed "this group sucks" in the middle of the group's fourth session. During the follow-up interview, the young man reflected on how surprised he was that I had not either thrown him out of the group or condemned him for his behavior: "I thought to myself, he's not yelling at me yet. After this (situation), you showed me you weren't utterly and completely incompetent" (Bein, 2008, p. 38).

Even higher praise than not being utterly and completely incompetent was given by another youth who remarked in a post-group interview: "After (that boy) said that and you dealt with it, I thought (this group) could be real cool" (Bein, 2008, p. 38).

Again, radical acceptance is not about taking an anything goes, laissez-faire approach. There are rules and boundaries, and sometimes there are consequences for out-of-bounds behavior. Clients learn that expectations for group or individual sessions exist in order to create an optimal environment for growth. What practitioner radical acceptance *does* provide clients is the sense that they will be supported and appreciated regardless of the "package" that he or she shows up in. That package includes historical behavior, nuanced present ways of being, and personal attributes relating to ethnicity/race, gender, sexual orientation, mental health challenges, and levels of engagement or cooperation with the counseling process.

Practitioner radical acceptance also provides a safe, less reactive environment. If practitioners radically accept their own arising emotions and thoughts, when limits are set or consequences are implemented, the client more likely experiences them as fairly and sincerely applied, not generated from reactivity. Sincerely and nonreactively facing our own (mental health practitioners') struggles models for clients the similar possibilities.

Should we become reactive, we may move toward (a) constructing a story regarding how unfit the client is for the program or the therapeutic endeavor; (b) engaging in a power struggle in order to put a "stop" to the behavior; and (c) confronting the client in order that she recognizes the folly of her ways, perhaps creating more client vulnerability than is necessary. Essentially, emotional reactivity takes practitioners out of Wise Mind. The only entrance back in is to notice, nonjudgmentally, that we are being reactive and finding a way to connect to the present moment where we and our clients reside.

Intention and Mindfulness Fueling Effective Practice

The capacity to maintain a strong back and soft front as well as to practice radical acceptance stems from three factors: (a) a well-developed intention to engage with clients in this manner; (b) the practice of mindfulness during our moment-to-moment interactions during sessions; and (c) the cultivation of mindfulness practice outside of sessions.

We outline for clients that practicing Wise Mind necessitates an *intention* to practice in this manner. Intention sets the ground for establishing commitment, remembering to invoke the skills, and setting a course for creating a life and life patterns that are different. As discussed in Chapter 2, intention is a bit different than a resolution. Intention points us toward a way of being, whereas resolutions tend to be framed as imposed outcomes to attain in order to improve ourselves. *We are fine just as we are*; we set intentions not so much for "self-improvement" but to live in accord with a greater sense of well-being and to make a positive impact.

Intention works for mental health practitioners in the same manner that it does for clients. Effective DBT-WR practice involves practitioner awareness of strong back and soft front, and anchoring our presence in our calm breath and radically accepting stance. If we do happen to become personally reactive, we remember to draw on our intention to take care of ourselves so as to maximize our presence and set a positive example of being able to flow with various emotions, situations, and thoughts.

Mindfulness is a core skill for DBT-WR clients. Clinician mindfulness in moment-to-moment work with clients sets the stage for providing these lessons. Koerner (2012) comments that "as a DBT therapist: in each interaction you practice observing, describing, and participating" (p. 202). Additionally, clinicians utilize mindfulness to practice "what works" (Koerner, 2012), which may involve letting go of judgments, settling into our breath, or responding actively and skillfully.

> The DBT therapist connects, again and again, with her client and her own experience, with open, spacious attention, noting and letting go of habitual judging, grasping, and avoiding. The therapist deliberately practices in

order to cultivate the qualities of mind to meet all experience with a welcoming, friendly stance, like the sun shining on all things equally. (Koerner, 2012, p. 203)

It is suggested that clinicians have some kind of mindfulness practice in order to meaningfully project the skills and to address, from experience, challenges that clients may have implementing them (Dimidjian & Linehan, 2003; Fulton, 2005; Koerner, 2012; Segal et al., 2002). In attempting to integrate mindfulness-based stress reduction (MBSR) principles for cognitive therapy addressing depression, Segal et al. (2002) discussed how their collective ambivalence about personally adopting a mindfulness practice was transformed:

The staff at the Stress Reduction Clinic had consistently emphasized the importance of instructors having their own meditation practice, and within minutes of meeting us, they asked about our personal commitment to the practice of mindfulness. We had now seen for ourselves the remarkable way they were able to embody a different relationship to the most intense distress and emotion in their patients. And we had seen the MBSR instructors going further in their work with negative affect than we had been able to do . . . within our therapist roles. We now saw more clearly how these two things were connected: that this ability to relate differently to negative affect came from having their own ongoing mindfulness practice, so that they might teach mindfulness out of their experience of it. *A vital part of what the MBSR instructor conveyed was his or her embodiment of mindfulness in interactions with the class.* (p. 56; italics mine)

The practitioner's mindfulness training may involve regular practice of short meditation periods (as little as 3 minutes) or yoga practice. As mentioned above, regular practice helps us embody mindfulness, and it gives us insight regarding struggles that clients may have with it. Additionally, clinicians' adopting our own practice universalizes the need to deeply connect with our internal process and to cultivate capacity to choose a path that is different from automatic pilot or emotional reactivity.

Use-of-Self With Challenging Clients and Circumstances

Challenging client or work contexts arise that may provoke clinician emotional reactivity and fight or flight fantasies or behavior. These situations are excellent practice opportunities, and we learn to approach them in this manner. Our commitment is to radically accept what is happening, stay mindful of our emotions and thoughts, and choose skillful responses that reduce our reactivity as well as keep us in effective relationship with clients.

One possible scenario is illustrative. During one group, one male client discussed how he was not sure whether any of this stuff would work for him. He had recently come out of prison and started using drugs again. As he sat in group, he mentioned how he felt like he was trying to get his head clear, and he was tired of people telling him what to do. I experienced his tone as aggressive toward me, but he was cordial with other group members. He spoke a fair amount; he was usually on topic, but it also seemed that he was competing for air time and sometimes veered off topic. I left the first group with feeling like the tent was big enough to work with him and the group and, though he would be challenging, believed that things would work out. He had even apologized to me as he left the group, in case, as he said, he was out of order.

During the next group, he was quite agitated. He made negative comments about people outside the group, which we had to contain, then took exception with something I said.

I had mentioned that my intention with them (the group members) was not to help them be "good clients"—meaning my attempts were not focused on helping them merely satisfy the agency rules and test clean (similar to the discussion in Chapter 3); instead, I was focused on helping them gain skills so they could feel more liberated in their lives. The client interpreted my words to mean that I did not care whether the group members did well in the program, so he asked, "What is the damn point of you being here?"

These kinds of moments are wonderful opportunities to put skills into practice. I settled into my seat, aware of my strong back and solid presence. I was mindful of the bit of fear that did arise, accompanied with thoughts like: "Am I going to lose control of the group?" "What can I say to help him see my intentions without sounding desperate?" "Is he going to step up his level of agitation?" Anchored in my breath, I empathized with his concern and let him know the point of my remarks. I stayed open-hearted to the degree that he at least wanted to make it through the group without feeling discouraged and activated, *and* I was undaunted enough by his remarks that we continued through the exercises.

As previously discussed regarding the teen group, some of the most profound experiences for group members can involve how situations like this are handled—*it is all part of the curriculum*. I scanned the room and noticed that no one was visibly shaken, though I knew that I would not be able to perceive everything, including some freeze responses. I decided, however, not to check in with everyone about feelings of safety in the group, believing that doing so would have stirred him up more. I also did not want to entertain personal thoughts of excluding him from returning after the break because, first, this chain of events would merely repeat for him what others had done in response to his behavior, and second, because his behavior did not so clearly "cross the line." There was also an opportunity for group learning that would be missed with merely excluding him.

As a metaphor for emotion regulation, a situation arose that stirred us up as a group. Acting on the group's behalf, I maintained my strong back while radically accepting what was occurring. I noticed my own level of activation, but did not move into fight–flight–freeze, instead acted skillfully to address the situation and move forward. All was apparently calm in the second half of the group. I said good-bye to the members as they left, then singled out the person who had confronted me and told him that "I am on your side." He countered that he did not need me, that he had God who was on his side, "that is all I need."

Again, this client had given me the gift of stirring me up, and thoughts and emotions concerning the group would intermittently arise until the next week when I would see him. At different times during the week, I noticed fantasies of having him leave the group as well as fantasies of not doing this group any longer. Being mindful of my states of agitation and of these mental fantasies helped me radically accept that this circumstance was challenging. I was able to accept and face this challenge—which included fear, insecurity about failing, and irritation—without lapsing into reactive postures such as finding ways to exclude the client.

In addition to maintaining my intention to use Wise Mind, be mindful of arising thoughts and emotions, and be skillful and nonreactive, I employed opposite action in dealing with the client the following week. Though, I was aware of thoughts to avoid making eye contact as I walked from the parking lot to the office, I acted in an opposite manner. I made eye contact and let myself experience my soft front for him in the form of our basic human connection. "Hey, it's great to see you today," I said sincerely. His response was similarly warm. I had mentally prepared to set limits and talk about each client's need to lessen their emotional charge before speaking in group, but this kind of discussion was not necessary.

In fact, the client's subsequent participation was thoughtful and transformative each group. I acknowledged times when he appeared overloaded, and sometimes we would take a breath for a while or tell a joke (soft front). When he stood up a couple of minutes before the group finished, I asked him to stay seated until the end of the group (strong back). I internally appreciated and openly acknowledged his enthusiasm and participation (soft front), then minutes later, I directed his focus back to the group member who was talking and away from the private conversation he was engaged in (strong back).

Personal practice of mindfulness, radical acceptance, and strong back/soft front skills helps practitioners integrate them while the session is unfolding in the here-and-now. Additionally, the practitioner's emotional self-regulation grounds the learning environment for each client. Being willing to enter murky, uncertain waters with a well-developed clinical use-of-self helps create an environment where clients are assured that: (a) the practitioner will address rather than deny arising issues; (b) respect from the practitioner will not be compromised by the *clinician's* reactivity; (c) the clinician will do everything possible to create a supportive, validating milieu where change and meaningful growth may occur; (d) the practitioner's radical acceptance of circumstances and people means an inclusive, tolerant environment where people can, with few exceptions, be themselves; and (e) the practitioner practices nondefensiveness.

Responding to Diversity as *Opportunity,* Not as Nuisance

Sometimes we, as clinicians, are wed to a story about who the clients are and how a session is going to unfold. Then we meet someone who has some cognitive challenges and struggles understanding the materials. Someone else has PTSD and is threatened by the "open field" of even the shortest mindfulness exercise period, but seems to do well chanting a phrase about being safe (e.g., "May I be safe, may I be okay"). Descriptions about "willfulness" are confusing and too abstract, but the entire group rallies around, embraces, and comprehends a group member's definition of willfulness—"do things my own fucking way." The lesson of the day does not focus on anxiety, but a group member walks in with unexplained terror, so we use the skills to help her deal with anxiety (of course, throwing off the "agenda").

Maintaining flexibility and consistently tuning into client needs provides the substantive foundation for inclusion. Not only are individual needs addressed and met, but clients learn the true nature of responsiveness. Diverse member needs and arising situations do not have to create a crisis for the practitioner within the session. Accommodation and spontaneity are balanced with structure in a manner where the container is not too rigid or too loose.

As one person's situation with anxiety is addressed, other people learn valuable lessons about how to address anxiety. The nonexplicit curriculum expands to additional elements such as "I can state my needs and they will be accepted, heard and taken seriously. I am not bad for having a problem today." Another part of the curriculum becomes, this group leader can hold what arises without pushing it away—parallel to the radical acceptance lessons that are integral in DBT-WR.

The accepting environment becomes one where clients increasingly take risks. The practitioner's *ethnographic curiosity* invites clients to grapple with their point of view and show up with their honest feelings and concerns (Bein, 2003). In another group, as mentioned earlier, a Latina client questioned whether the DBT-WR lessons were an attempt to teach her how to be White. The attempt here is to understand how she came to this thought and to engage in a mutually respectful dialogue where each of us can emerge with new understandings.

As we engage in this manner, it may make sense to adjust language and explanations. Where, in one instance, broad spiritual language seems inclusive because it opens the door for people with less formalized religious beliefs, in another instance it seems overly nondescript and too "new age-ey." Where some people appreciate the notion of radical acceptance and sense how it connects, for them, with 12-step philosophy, other people are repelled by the language of acceptance because—no matter how much explained otherwise—it implies approval of acts that are not to be approved. These sentiments become the basis of modifying language and offering culturally competent terms such as *radical nonreactivity* or *radical showing up*.

Evidence–Based Practice

The ongoing incorporation of clinical expertise and nuanced client needs within an existing practice modality does *not* contaminate evidence-based practice. In fact, these nuanced essentials, along with common factors research, emphasizing the importance of the client–practitioner relationship, enhance the substantive viability of an evidence-based practice (EBP) (Littell, 2010). In other words, practice evolution and dynamic client–practitioner dialogue about what is understandable, meaningful, and helpful may not only bring viability to an EBP, but adjustments may be necessary in order for the practice to have feasibility.

Arguing otherwise means advancing not EBP per se, but *evidence-based treatment* (EBT), which "restricts practice [and] is the creation of orthodoxy" (Littell, 2010, p. 186).

The guiding principles of inclusion and mental health recovery demand that dynamic client input, creative practitioner methods for client inclusiveness, and thoughtful, dedicated practitioner use-of-self need to be part of the therapeutic package.

The central limitation of EBP is the tendency to reduce rather than amplify meaning. The more central EBP becomes, the more decontextualized, objectified and divested of meaning the patient becomes. (Slade, 2009, p. 139)

This book's task is to consider DBT in a manner that clinicians for years have considered cognitive-behavioral therapy—a powerful, evidence-based technology that may be dynamically applied for diverse populations and settings. This DBT-WR approach endeavors to work from DBT's foundation of evidenced success and offer possibilities across various settings and client situations.

Practitioner Nondefensiveness

In order to bolster the acceptance/validation portion of the dialectic, practitioners need to personally demonstrate that regardless of client behavior, client thoughts about the helping process, and client judgments or emotional responses to the practitioner, they will remain steadfast in their overall acceptance of the client or consumer. Practitioner nondefensiveness goes a long way toward achieving that result. Practitioners who are highly attached to outcome, either because they struggle psychologically with mediating demands of the service context or because their ego is identified with the results, are more vulnerable to becoming defensive with clients.

Nondefensiveness models nonreactivity and emotion regulation for clients. For many reasons clients engage in provocative behavior or make controversial or upsetting comments that may stir you as the practitioner. The origin of these client actions may involve (a) testing you to see whether you will accept them regardless of their conduct; (b) assessing whether their style of thinking and ways of being could be integrated into the treatment philosophy and context; (c) expecting failure and rejection and setting up conditions to promote this result; (d) being in a precontemplative stage within the change process; (e) having an oppositional personality style or general "willfulness" (that may especially be fueled in a group setting); (f) being emotionally activated and, perhaps, threatened by either the treatment context, a particular event that happened in the course of treatment, or the practitioner's personal characteristics or behavior; or (g) not imagining that the treatment suggestions could work for them.

Staying true to emotion regulation work in the DBT-WR tradition, our primary task is not to cognitively "get to the bottom" of why the client's behavior is happening. We start with noticing our own arising emotions and thoughts, we accept the circumstances and our internal process, and we commit to nonreactivity and being present for the client. We may lean into our strong back, take a deep breath, and find solidity and calmness in the swirl of emotion and activity. We may have to establish limits and help the client become grounded if the behavior is escalating and/or is threatening to others. From this strong-back base, we engage our soft front to curiously explore the client's struggles or dissonance.

Our defensiveness would interfere with these processes. We may act from emotional wounds, disappointment, or anger and not only enhance the client–practitioner divide, but also unintentionally model for clients that the way to deal with difficult emotions is to become defensive, which is to say *reactive*.

Defensive practitioner behavior also enhances the split between what is preached and what is observed ("do as I say, not as I do"). However, practitioner willingness to *be with* challenging circumstances and not react lets clients see that you are walking the walk. When clients gain a glimpse of some of your own past struggles in walking this walk, they appreciate that nondefensiveness and emotion regulation is a process, and that you, the practitioner, were not magically imbued with this capacity. This kind of practitioner self-disclosure is encouraged in the DBT tradition (Koerner, 2012).

Practitioner nondefensiveness contributes to overall feelings of safety within the helping environment. Many clients, particularly those with a trauma background, are on alert for practitioner behavior that seems attacking or rejecting. Some may even attempt to stimulate these responses, stemming from a sense that there is more control in creating a scenario that ends in practitioner anger or rejection than in anxiously anticipating that at some random, nonpredictable moment the shoe will drop. Staying the course of nondefensiveness and reactivity, though unfamiliar at first for some clients, inevitably helps them settle into a feeling that the environment is safe.

Finally, safety in the treatment setting combined with practitioner openness and nondefensiveness create conditions to collaboratively navigate the environment and work on client issues. Clients learn the precious interpersonal lessons of skillfully discussing their needs rather than acting out frustrations or assuming their needs will not be addressed. If the therapist or practitioner is nonreactively responding to the client, then the working agreement becomes the practitioner's commitment to sincerely address concerns "in exchange for" the client's commitment to honestly explore change.

Language of Invitation

Spending a week with Jon Kabat-Zinn was intensive exposure to the art form of the *language of invitation*. This kind of language approach is congruent with motivational interviewing and carries an implicit message—desired in DBT-WR—that the client is radically accepted as she is *right now* and that she is being invited to consider new possibilities. Practitioner judgment regarding client behavior as well as overexuberant and sometimes invalidating pushing is less likely to emerge if the practitioner has cultivated the intention to use inviting language. Underlying the language of invitation is a spirit of radical acceptance and of opening doors slowly. While the client is experiencing some form of control regarding pacing, she decides whether and to what extent she will cross the threshold and take steps toward change. *I am wondering what some of your (the reader's) objections would be to these kinds of conversations. I am sure your objections are understandable and well thought out. To what extent would you be willing to experiment using this kind of language and then see what worked for you and what did not work.* Get it?

Use-of-Self Summary

Your thoughtful, aware, and heartfelt use-of-self is a powerful vehicle for delivering DBT-WR to your clients. Core concepts like radical acceptance, Wise Mind, and mindfulness are not as easily understood as, say, identifying a cognitive distortion (CBT). In addition to the delivered content (see next chapter), clients experience and learn DBT-WR lessons through their here-and-now experience of you, the practitioner, as well as the container that you establish. As you attend to these use-of-self issues, DBT-WR will come more from your own Wise Mind rather than from a detached intellectual understanding. May you enjoy the journey.

Six

Lessons and Activities: Dialectical Behavior Therapy for Wellness and Recovery

Principles for Using Lessons

Lessons are designed for building proficiency in how to non-reactively deal with emotions and thoughts, to accept/face arising situations and internal processes, to improve the moment and/or access the bigger picture (also called "expanding the moment"), and to live with greater self-compassion and wellness. After the initial lesson, which focuses on the connection between mindfulness and neuroplasticity, Lesson 2 provides a guiding, visual framework that anchors all the subsequent DBT-WR lessons and activities. Special attention is paid to clients maintaining the *intention* to access Wise Mind, which is the mind that is not hijacked by emotion, has balance, and has problem-solving capacity. In Lessons 2 through 9, the session is formatted to conduct an opening check-in regarding the client's recent (i.e., since the prior session) Wise Mind work. The term *Wise Mind* is repeated throughout DBT-WR and serves as an anchor point for clients.

In general, the Wise Mind is accepting, mindful, nonimpulsive, self-compassionate, and thoughtful. The Wise Mind maintains stability in the face of making mistakes and, perhaps most important, *seeks self-care in the midst of distress*. The Wise Mind is sufficiently mindful of one's internal process; it motivates the individual to step outside the fray and observe what is happening, and it provides the foundation for living in balance and moment-to-moment wellness. Clients, however, will come to their own understandings of Wise Mind, and it seems preferable to let their insights evolve, rather than attempting to impose a precise Wise Mind definition.

DBT-WR process steps are offered to clients in Lesson 2 and may be helpful to summarize here; they accompany the Wise Mind figure that is provided in Lesson 2.

Step 1: Developing the intention to live in Wise Mind to enhance wellness. Intention relates to inclining the mind toward nonreactivity and present-focused awareness as well as to cultivating commitment.

Step 2: Accepting what arises. That means noticing emotions, thoughts, and situations without reacting. Some people prefer other language in lieu of *accepting*, such as *radical nonreactivity*, *facing what is*, or *showing up for what is*. All these terms mean facing the truth of what is happening. Tuning into our breath helps in this process.

Step 3: Improving the moment. Sometimes just accepting things as they are improves the moment. Other times, accepting is only a first step; something else needs to occur in order to improve the moment, such as letting go and releasing, seeking support, or engaging in healthy forms of soothing or healthy distraction.

Step 4: Expanding the moment/accessing the bigger picture. Spirituality may be accessed to help deal with troubling emotions, thoughts, or situations. For some, that means connecting to a higher power and letting the higher power or the universe "have" your problems. Others may explore their understanding regarding their deeper purpose in the world or seek paths or deeper connections beyond the conventional small self.

Step 5: Generating self-compassion for support. Self-care and nurturance is enhanced through accessing one's patient, loving, and compassionate self. Tapping into self-compassion enhances personal wellness and recovery.

Improve the Moment: Language and Meaning

Linehan (1993) conceptualizes *improve the moment* as a pragmatic skill for distress tolerance. In the midst of difficulty, the commitment to improve the moment taps into personal awareness that emotional well-being can be improved through (a) engaging in positive actions, (b) changing thought processes or cognitive appraisals about present situations, or (c) creating meaning or deeper connection.

This book's DBT-informed model emphasizes improve the moment as a core strategy because its utilization enhances one's on-the-spot capacity for creating enhanced wellness and recovery. The notion of improve the moment empowers us to take note of and accept (face) our present state of affairs—psychologically, sociologically, and spiritually. Mindful awareness of our difficult emotional states and circumstances provide a base to move forward (improve), instead of feeling choice-less, victimized, and reactive. Equipped with the notion that we can *improve the moment*, we consistently remain aware that we are empowered. Sometimes clearly seeing what is happening, not fighting against reality (radically accepting), and providing self-compassion are enough to improve the moment. Paradoxically, in these instances, we improve the moment through surrendering to what is, realizing that there is not much we can do other than to feel what we are feeling and to hold ourselves with self-compassion.

Other times, we realize that "things could be better"; thus, we improve our emotional state, change our immediate behavior, and, perhaps, modify our cognitive approach. We also may take steps, both subtle and profound, to change life conditions. When we sense that we can "improve the moment," we may decide to take a shower rather than stay in bed and perseverate, we may decide to visualize troublesome thoughts floating away on a cloud, or we may decide to skillfully navigate interpersonal situations rather than feeling personally victimized or emotionally reactive. Improving the moment means taking a step toward a greater sense of well-being.

People may prefer the language "respond to the moment"—discussed earlier in the book—in lieu of improve the moment. In essence, all we can do is respond. We ultimately have no control over whether the *response* leads to improvement; therefore, clients may wish to consult Figure 2.1, page 23. *Responding to the moment* removes the measuring stick, implicit for some, with improve-the-moment language. Finally, responding to the moment seems to be more consonant with the DBT-WR process. Within a personally mindful and self-compassionate environment and spurred by a personal intention for wellness, the individual *responds* to arising events and phenomena (including emotions and thoughts). "Improve," on the other hand, implies a betterment of outcomes over which we actually have little control.

Continuing this line of thought, we can critique the linguistic construction of "improve the moment." Contemplating its nature, we notice that the moment just *is*—it arises and passes. How can it actually be improved? Being mindful and accepting of the moment and applying an intention to making things better—perhaps more accurately—means that we are endeavoring to improve the *next* moment.

Despite its flaws, the phrase "improve the moment" offers hope, clarity, and direction for people seeking enhanced emotional regulation and wellness. Where "respond to the moment" appears neutral, improve the moment points toward possibilities for developing on-going resilience and wellness and for soothing and coping with arising emotional distress. Hence, improve the moment is chosen for the DBT-WR scheme presented to clients.

Overall, improve the moment and other constructs are grappled with and language is sometimes modified as per the client's cultural, linguistic, and cognitive proclivities. Ultimately, a construct is a representation or idea about reality; it is not reality, itself. We embrace the dialectic between the power and compelling nature of constructs with the need to hold them lightly and allow for personal interpretation and ascription of value.

Session Structure and Flow

Based on the recovery and use-of-self principles discussed throughout this book, it may be desirable to flatten the client–practitioner hierarchy and be aware of the dialectic between a well-presented, organized lesson and a lesson that has spontaneity and is structured, to some degree, around client input and flow of the session. Individuals in one-on-one sessions may proceed rapidly through posed questions offered in each lesson, and writing down responses within the lessons may make sense. Questions or activities that are not covered in an individual session could be given as "homework."

In group settings, there may be significant energy around addressing a particular item. As long as it is not off-task, it may be beneficial to build off the momentum of the group and spend significant time on one item. You will often find that follow-up questions within a lesson have already been addressed if you are fortunate enough to have an animated, in-depth discussion. After a thorough exploration, it is acceptable to deal with follow-up items within the lesson and say, "it seems like we have already addressed that one," or maybe "let's move forward and look at another area now."

Overall, the lesson materials are meant as an aide to address vital issues; rigidly adhering to completing all items either by plowing through too rapidly or meticulously covering everything interferes with creating a dynamic treatment environment. It may make sense to spend more than one session with a particular lesson.

As mentioned, Lessons 2 through 9 begin with a check-in regarding how clients used their Wise Mind since the last session. You may want to continue that ritual through later sessions, especially if you have an open-ended group and there were members who joined the group near session 9. It is also helpful to show both individual and group clients the Wise Mind figure at the beginning of the session (perhaps at the beginning of each one). Some people are extraordinarily visual and will study this figure closely. The figure depicts emotional wellness in a memorable, useful map.

You may want to attend to three other issues related to session structure. First, some clients receive more benefit if there are at least some opportunities for writing. In a group setting, this sometimes evens the playing field with more verbally active members. Clients get a few minutes to consider their thoughts and then write. When they are called on, there is something on the paper. If literacy skills are limited, clients could be encouraged to offer a symbol that will help them remember what they would want to say; the papers do not have to be collected.

Second, you may want to consider a 3-minute breathing meditation, walking exercise, or eating exercise as a regular part of the session. Some clients who are not inclined to do these exercises regularly on their own still testify as to how they remembered an in-group exercise, and, in a moment of distress, utilized it. This kind of client experience is more likely if there are regular, in-group opportunities for practice.

We will talk about the spirit of conducting these exercises just below.

Third, clients benefit from some form of "checking out" at the end of the session, which could mean evaluating the session or practitioner (Duncan, Miller, & Sparks, 2004). This evaluation could be formal, or could involve a response to the question, "What happened for you during this session?" In a larger group, this allows for a response from every member, and, in general, may provide valuable feedback for you, the practitioner.

Homework

There is a two-page, easy-to-fill-out "Log for Daily Living" that is provided at the end of Lesson 5. The log corresponds to the main tracking points for clients and has value for those who diligently complete it. (Another copy of the "Log for Daily Living" is provided in the Appendix.) Generally, people experience greater progress if they are systematically thinking about and implementing lessons and strategies; completing the log encourages this behavior. However, some people are averse to anything that sounds like homework—no matter how you couch it—and it may not be productive to hold one's feet to the fire or engage in a power struggle regarding out-of-session work. As mentioned in the book, I have seen people do excellent DBT-WR work, but they did it on their own terms and eschewed formal assignments. Having a strong back about homework (see Chapter 5) may help establish conditions for client growth, or it may unnecessarily push someone out.

There are a few questions (Lesson 6) that prompt a discussion regarding attitudes about homework. Although the questions are simple and closed-ended, they are framed so as to facilitate a nonblaming, ethnographically oriented discussion. These homework-related questions may be interjected during other lessons.

Approaching the Lessons With a Light-Hearted Spirit

You may guide a mindfulness exercise through a word-by-word reading of the steps outlined in Lesson 2. You could then experiment with leaving the steps behind and trying to ad lib. As you begin any mindfulness exercise, you always want to encourage the client(s) to notice self-judgments but to let them go. We (both clients and practitioners) inevitably evaluate or rate how "well" we are doing, and that kind of running monologue sometimes drowns out our actual experience.

The best way for you to encourage your client's efforts to nonjudgmentally and self-compassionately observe what is arising is for you, the practitioner, to embody lightheartedness and drop your personal achievement fixations. You do not need to pretend that you always know what you are doing or that you are the champion 3-minute mindfulness leader. Your capacity to ride with mistakes, relax with what is, and maintain your humanness represent powerful lessons for your clients.

Lesson 1: Mindfulness and the Brain

Learning About the Brain

The amygdala is referred to as an alarm center. It mobilizes energy for survival including our reactive fight, flight, or freeze responses. The amygdala creates fiery responses and may cause the stress hormone cortisol to spike. Although high levels of cortisol may help us run away or scare off an attacker, they create the following problems:

➤ Chronic stress

➤ Becoming overreactive, angry, and explosive about situations

➤ Feeling out of balance with our emotions

➤ Feeling like it is hard to feel calm and to soothe ourselves

➤ Having difficulty making decisions that are helpful to us and to those around us

The good news is that we can alter our brain! Mindfulness is the key.

Through a process called neuroplasticity we can actually change how our brain functions and create greater wellness in our lives. We get there through being able to observe our brain and see how our brain works. *We actually begin to have a relationship with our brain.*

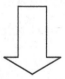

When we have a careful, mindful focus of attention, we enhance activity in the part of the brain that we want to be in: the **prefrontal cortex.**

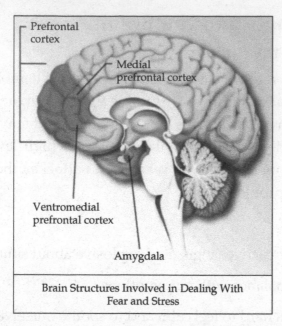

Medial prefrontal– Monitor behavior/ prevent undesirable action (Gehring & Fencsik, 2001)
Ventromedial prefrontal–Regulating emotions; deals with fear, uncertainty in making decisions (Blair, 2008)

Brain Structures Involved in Dealing With
Fear and Stress

Figure from National Institute of Mental Health, *Post-traumatic stress disorder research fact sheet*. [Data file] Retrieved from http://www.nimh.nih.gov/health/publications/post-traumatic-stress-disorder-research-fact-sheet/index.shtml Used with permission. (For further information on the relationship between the amygdala and the prefrontal cortex see Siegel, 2010).

Mindfulness for a Healthy Mind

Practicing Mindfulness   Mindfulness means open awareness to the present moment. The following steps are part of a mindfulness practice session. **You will engage in this practice later.**

➤ Sit quietly and comfortably.

➤ Take a deep breath and release some of the tension as you exhale.

➤ Breathe naturally.

➤ Notice when your mind wanders and let go of thoughts or feelings that arise.

➤ Come back to your breath when you notice you have drifted away.

➤ Let go of judgments about your performance; you are doing it perfectly no matter what your experience is like.

People have various ideas about mindfulness that may enhance or interfere with their engagement. You may believe that you are not capable of sitting quietly and observing your thoughts or you may believe that if you sit quietly, troublesome thoughts will come up and you will be worse off. Here are a few things to consider that may change the way you think about mindfulness.

1. Mindfulness is about creating peace in your life. There is no right way to do it. It is natural and completely okay to either not want to do the short exercise, to think the exercise is stupid, to have fears about the exercise, or, conversely, to be hopeful about mindfulness.

2. If you are already noticing your thoughts and feelings about mindfulness, you are *already doing mindfulness*. The 3-minute mindfulness exercise represents a preparation for practicing mindfulness in the rest of your life and for enhancing your Wise Mind.

3. Religious traditions around the world—including Christianity—engage in practices and contemplations that enhance our connection to the Universe and our sense of peace. People of all religious traditions practice mindfulness and people who do not consider themselves spiritual or religious practice mindfulness.

4. During a short mindfulness exercise, you have the opportunity to be generous and kind to yourself. Ideas will arise involving judgments of yourself regarding how well you are doing. The trick is to notice the judgments as stories or thoughts that can be released. *You will eventually learn to "stare down" judgments of yourself that you carry around with you all the time!!!*

Client Activity

What are you aware of *right now* (thoughts, impressions, feelings, questions) regarding mindfulness exercises? Please know that whatever is in your awareness is okay.

_____

_____

Client Activity

Do a 3-minute breathing activity (meditation) using the steps above. The mind will get distracted from the breath. The idea is to bring it back to the breath. Whether you are getting glimpses of focusing on your breath, learning how to bring your attention back to your breath, noticing what is arising, or simply being distracted most of the time:

No matter how you are doing, you are doing fine!!

Be compassionate with yourself.

Motivation and Reasons for Practicing Mindfulness

Mindfulness practice helps you be less reactive. The mindful mind is not hijacked by arising emotions, past or present events, or worrisome thoughts. Mindfulness actually **rewires the brain** so that more activity takes place in the prefrontal cortex.

The frontal areas of your brain help with:

Regulating mood

Emotional balance

Insight

Empathy

Fear modulation

Trauma

You may have had to deal with traumatic experiences in your life and your brain put you on high alert so that you could be safe and prepared to fight or flee. As a result,

You are in fight–flight–freeze mode; you may feel anxious, reactive, and angry.

Client Activity

HOW IS YOUR BRAIN REACTIVE?

What are times when you are quick to get *angry,* feel **anxious,** or feel like you want to *avoid* people or situations?

Angry Situations (Fight)

1. _____

2. _____

Anxious Situations (Freeze)

1. _____

2. _____

Avoidant Situations (Flight)

1. _____

2. _____

Using your *Wise Mind* means to be less reactive, more calm, and less in conflict with the world—how much would you want to live that way?

_____

_____

_____

Lesson 2: Facing Emotions and Thoughts and Improving the Moment

[*First, check in regarding client recent use of Wise Mind; then, refer to the Wise Mind figure to discuss improving the moment.*]

You become less reactive and feel more effective in the world when you can *work with* distressing thoughts and emotions that arise. The best way to work with them is to see difficult thoughts and emotions for what they are—accept them—and develop a strategy to deal with them. **The thoughts and emotions do not have to take over your life!**

Strategies for Facing Difficulties and Improving the Moment

Let's cover all the steps first and then look more closely at the important points. These steps are displayed pictorially on the next page. (A full-page handout/presentation version of the Wise Mind figure is available in the Appendix.)

Step 1: Develop the *intention* that you want to be more calm, less reactive, and more joyful about living in the world. *You need to live in your Wise Mind to accomplish this*. Your Wise Mind is more effective and balanced and is not overtaken by strong emotions like anger and despair.

Step 2: *Accept* what arises for you. That means notice your emotions, your thoughts, and the situation you are in without reacting. If you have trouble with the word *accept*, you can use other terms: *radical nonreactivity, facing what is, showing up for what is*. Accepting means facing the truth of what is happening. Tuning into our breath helps.

Step 3: *Improve the moment*. Sometimes just accepting things as they are improves the moment, because you no longer feel that you *have to* do something, or because accepting thoughts and emotions allows them to have less of a hold on you. Other times accepting is only a first step, and you will need to do something else to improve the moment. These strategies are listed and usually involve one of these forms: letting go and releasing, seeking support, or engaging in either healthy soothing or healthy distraction.

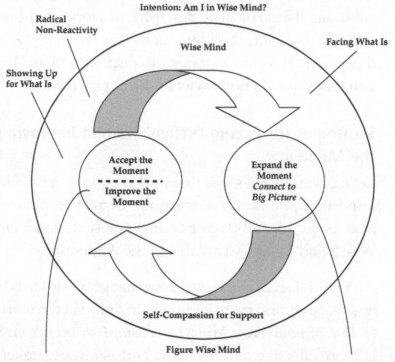

Intention: Am I in Wise Mind?

Radical Non-Reactivity

Wise Mind

Facing What Is

Showing Up for What Is

Accept the Moment
- - - - - - - -
Improve the Moment

Expand the Moment
Connect to Big Picture

Self-Compassion for Support

Figure Wise Mind

Being with breath & not reacting.
Letting go of judgments.
Engaging in what soothes/I enjoy.
Mindfulness—one thing at a time.
Friend to self & support from others.
Grounding self & embracing safety.
Distraction from distress.
Effective speech & interpersonal skills.
Awareness of primary & secondary emotions.
Doing what is needed & not getting hooked.

My "job" is about healing & freedom.
What does my higher power want for me?
I belong on the planet.
Life is more than this moment of suffering.
What is my deepest purpose?
Courage to tell the truth to self.

Step 4: *Expand the moment.* You may connect in some way to your spirituality to help you deal with troubling emotions, thoughts, or situations. For some that means connecting to your higher power and giving your problems away to your higher power or "the universe." Others may explore their commitment to their deeper purpose in the world. Sometimes this deeper purpose relates to the kind of person you want to be or thinking about how you may inspire others through your life or recovery.

Step 5: *Self-compassion for support.* This is not so much a "step" but refers to the way you want to be as you do this work. Continue to find the patient, loving, and compassionate part of yourself that appreciates who you are and recognizes that you will not be perfect. If you mindfully tap into self-compassion your life will be happier.

Client Activity

One element that makes a difference in **improving the moment** is your willingness and intention to attempt this work. When you apply **intention** to your everyday life, you begin to feel like you can create a life worth living. Some people say that intention includes effort and focus. **How would you define intention?**

_____

_____

Please be honest about how much you have the intention to **improve the moment?**

_____

_____

What are some things that may get in the way of having a strong intention?

_____

_____

Radical Acceptance

You may notice that being **mindful** of the moment is connected to nonreactivity or acceptance. **Nonreactivity** means not getting so emotionally intense right away and not jumping to a response that we may later regret.

Acceptance is similar. It means completely facing what is happening in the moment. Acceptance does not say we have to agree with what is happening or approve of it. We just have to realize that, yes, this is what is going on.

When you think about it, **radical acceptance** helps us **see clearly**. We are not so caught up in our emotions or the way that we would like things to be. We take a breath and think to ourselves that everything in the universe has led up to this moment—and here it is!!

Radical acceptance does not mean we are soft or passive.

Radical acceptance does not mean we approve of what is happening.

When someone is treating us badly, we radically accept this is happening. We do not deny it. That means we can *skillfully* **respond to the moment**.

Radical acceptance does mean that we deal with reality rather than fighting against reality.

We radically accept our own thoughts, feelings, or situations that arise. This acceptance creates **calmness** around what we are thinking, feeling, or facing in the world. When we are calm, our thoughts, emotions, or life circumstances do not pull us on a train of intense anger, despair, or rumination. If we happen to get on that train, we radically accept we are there and get ourselves off.

Which radical acceptance statements work the best for you:

➤ Everything has led up to this moment right now.

➤ I cannot change the past; I can only notice the moment and respond in the present.

➤ I can radically accept that it is hard to radically accept.

➤ I sense my higher power has a plan; it is my job to become a willing participant.

➤ Radical acceptance of myself and others will create more peace in my life.

➤ Radical acceptance means acceptance of everything. I may still be angry and resentful and act like a jerk. I accept that.

➤ Radical acceptance is about not judging and radically accepting myself when I am judging.

Which of these statements work for you, or do you prefer another?

_____

Please say why you made your choice.

_____

_____

Discuss how you think radical acceptance makes positive change more likely.

_____

_____

_____

Some people are hesitant to embrace radical acceptance because it means they would become less angry. What do you think about that?

_____

Radical acceptance gives you the clarity to skillfully **improve the moment**. Please look at the ways that you improve the moment over these next few days.

—— Client Activity ——

ACTIVITY: THE POWER OF RADICAL ACCEPTANCE

Close your eyes partially or fully. Tune into your slow, steady breath. Imagine that right now—**in this moment**—you are absolutely perfect, being just who you are. You sense that you radically accept yourself. Sense your calmness. Radically accept the thoughts that arise—maybe "no way," "this is BS," or "I like this"—and return to the breath. Notice and radically accept the emotions that arise, and return to the breath.

In this moment ➜ nothing to do

—— Client Activity ——

Later sessions will explore ways to improve the moment in more depth. For now, feel free to note down times over this next week when you were stirred up with intense thoughts or feelings. How much did you become mindful and accept that you were having these thoughts and feelings? What did you do to **improve the moment**, which means to take care of yourself so that you did not stay upset?

Day	Intense Emotions and Thoughts	Did you Accept/ Come Face-to-Face with Emotions?	How did you *Improve the Moment?*

Lesson 3: Dealing With Judgments

[First, check in regarding client recent use of Wise Mind; then, refer to the Wise Mind figure to discuss improving the moment.]

Judgments

Judgments are thoughts that we have about ourselves or others that we often believe are true. Judgments help us stay stuck and paralyzed in our own lives. The goal is to mindfully **notice** the judgment, **accept** that it is there, and then **let it go.**

Examples of Self-Judgment

"I'm no good." "I can't do this." "I am a bad person for . . . ."
Identify two judgments that you have about yourself

1. _____

2. _____

A common strategy is to counter the judgments with an argument about how the judgment is wrong. This is called a cognitive approach. An example of this would be to convert a judgment from something negative to something positive:

I'm a no good loser $\Longrightarrow$ **I am a good person**

Sometimes this strategy works, but many times it does not. That is because whether you think you are a loser or a good person, *you are still involved in judging yourself!* As long as you keep judging yourself, you will flip back and forth between something positive and something negative.

The idea is to let go of your judgments

Using mindfulness, we learn about how to witness judgments for what they are. Judgments are thoughts, not facts. As we witness them and do not engage with them, we are in a better position to let them go.

"Oh, there's that judgment again. . . ."

Client Activity

Choose one of the two self-judgments that you wrote about yourself to do this activity.

Close your eyes partially or fully—whatever feels best—and let your breath deepen. Let the self-judgment you chose enter the mind and see if you can look at the judgment as a collection of words that no longer represents who you really are.

See what it is like to release the judgment.
Put your attention back on your breath.
You can slowly open your eyes fully.

Another way to think about a judgment is to consider it a "story." [Some people really like this approach.] Often in the day, you spend time telling a story about yourself. You talk about how well you are doing; how much you deserve or don't deserve something; how good or bad of a person you are; and so on.

Think about the story that you tell yourself about *you*.

_____

_____

_____

What would it be like to notice and accept the story, then DROP IT?

_____

_____

Two Other Areas for Judgments:

Judgments about others

Judgments about having judgments

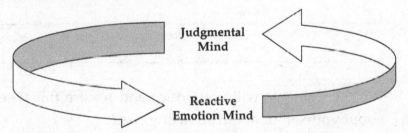

Emotional states/responses that arise from a judgmental place are not from WISE MIND.

Strategies for Judgments

- See judgments for what they are—NOTICE!!
  They are not the "truth." They are a story about reality.

- Accept the judgment as a judgment.

- Let the judgment go.
  → _Give to Higher Power_
  → _Let it drift away on a cloud_
  → _Breathe it out_

Accept the Moment/Improve the Moment

Letting go of judgments is an *improve the moment* strategy that helps us stay connected to the present moment. If we dwell in judgments about ourselves or others, we experience *our thoughts* about what is happening rather than what is *actually* happening itself. If we spend a lot of time dwelling in our judgments, **we miss our life in the present moment**.

How much do negative judgments about yourself interfere with your self-compassion?

_____

_____

How much would it be helpful to drop some judgments about other people?

_____

_____

What judgments will you notice and release this week—either about yourself or about someone else?

_____

_____

Lesson 4: Expanding the Moment

[First, check in regarding client recent use of Wise Mind; then, refer to the Wise Mind figure to discuss expanding the moment.]

Bigger Picture Strategies

Letting go of judgments of ourselves and appreciating our uniqueness helps us appreciate ourselves, *just as we are*. Sometimes it is helpful to expand the moment—that is, find a way to tap into a force or belief system that contains nurturance or self-compassion. Doing this work helps us hold the day-to-day struggles and challenges.

I **belong on the planet** is a realization we may arrive at when we contemplate our value.

➤ How much do you believe that you belong on the planet?

➤ What negative judgments have you had to overcome in order to believe that you belong on the planet? (Another way to think of belonging on the planet is: God has a plan for me.)

➤ In what way, if any, does your sense of belonging on the planet come from your belief in a higher power or your sense of something spiritual? Some people prefer to think of their deepest purpose and the source of that purpose.

➤ How much do you believe that you are a precious human being?

➤ What kinds of experiences have you had that give you a sense of your inner beauty or your importance to the world?

Client Activity

Which of these following practices is something that you already engage in? Which of these practices could you engage in more regularly?

Wise Mind—Expand the Moment Practice	Already Do This	Will Do More Often
Take a deep breath and step back from the situation		
Find a way to experience love for myself		
Connect to hopeful thoughts or places in my mind		
Give problems to my higher power		
Experience deep appreciation for the way I have overcome a lot in my life		
Pray		
Meditate / 3-minute breathing space		
Attend a 12-step meeting		
Let myself imagine being loved by God (the universe)		
Act with intention to make myself/another happy[1] (see page 175)		
Emphasize the journey over setbacks that may occur		
Other bigger picture practice ➜		

Expand-the-Moment Practices

Our connection to the "bigger picture" is enhanced through regular practices reminding us how our life is bigger than our day-to-day problems. When we are in a dark tunnel and life seems as though there is nothing but suffering and negativity, we use Wise Mind to put our struggles into perspective. Consult with the Wise Mind figure to see the place of expand the moment.

[1]We must make the important distinction between making ourselves happy and seeking temporary pleasure. What is the distinction in your mind?

_____

_____

When you are feeling low or "are in a dark tunnel," what is a good Wise Mind approach for you? In other words, how do you help yourself feel better in a bigger picture (spiritual) way when you are not feeling well?

_____

_____

Many people report that engaging in rituals help them feel more connected to their higher power or to sacred life rhythms. Some of these rituals may be very simple, like enjoying a cup of tea at night, and some may be more formal like making a sign of the cross before eating, meditating in the morning, or praying.

Some of us feel that rituals are oppressive or are not liberating for them. How much do you feel this way?

_____

_____

Can you imagine the reasons that daily rituals or yearly celebrations are important for people? What has been important for you? (Some of the patterns may be visiting family members once a year or celebrating a holiday.)

_____

_____

Despite our history or background with rituals, what kind of rituals or patterns of living can we imagine bringing into our lives?

_____

_____

Over this next week, please do the following:

Maintain a regular practice of engaging in a 3-minute meditation. This effort builds your mindfulness capacity.

And *experiment* with engaging in one bigger picture practice.

Expand the moment when you are facing difficult emotions or situations: Ask your higher power for help, assure yourself about the bigger journey, settle into your calm breath, etc.

OR

Search for and implement a consistent practice in your life (every day, once a week . . .) that helps connect you regularly to something bigger than your personal concerns and worries.

What do you think is the likelihood that you will do these assignments? *Let's Discuss.*

Lesson 5: Dealing With Difficult Times

Distress Tolerance Plan

[First, check in regarding client recent use of Wise Mind; then, refer to the Wise Mind figure to briefly discuss improving the moment and expanding the moment.]

We have experienced some difficult times in the past. Sometimes our strategies for dealing with what happened were helpful and we pulled through okay; other times we either did not have strategies or the way we dealt with our situation made things worse.

What are the ways you usually deal with things when you are in the middle of difficult times?

_____

_____

How helpful are your ways of coping with difficulty?

_____

_____

Soothing

Soothing ourselves is a way to take care of ourselves and to take care of our emotional lives. When we are *mindful of the moment* and tune into our emotions, we sense that we are angry or in some distress. We *accept* that this is happening to us, and then we need to *improve the moment.*

Soothing is a way of calming the intensity of our emotions. In the hot Southeast Asian jungles, people pour a cup of cool water over their heads and imagine that the water is compassion.

When we soothe ourselves, we reinforce the intention to live a life worth living and to take the steps we need to have ourselves be safe. Sometimes just taking one step in the direction of taking care of ourselves is powerful.

What are things that you can do to feel soothed (and perhaps slightly happy) when times are difficult? This is your Distress Tolerance Plan.

Client Activity

DISTRESS TOLERANCE PLAN

1. _____

2. _____

3. _____

4. _____

5. _____

What makes the strategies in this plan more helpful than ways you have dealt with distress in the past?

_____

_____

How much does staying in the moment help you to deal with your distress?

_____

_____

What kind of situation creates the most suffering for you?

_____

_____

How do you use an **expanding-the–moment**, bigger picture approach when times are difficult?

_____

_____

Aside from your distress tolerance plan, are there ways that you can approach these situations so **you will not end up in a crisis or emotional turmoil?**

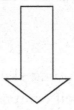

How Can I Prevent Intense Emotional Turmoil ?

Client Activity

- Start with the *intention* that this exercise may be meaningful for you.
- If you need to acknowledge and speak about how you don't think these kind of exercises work, please do so.
- Engage in the mindfulness exercise of pouring compassion over your head.
- You may imagine compassion in the form of light and ease.
- Proceed slowly as the compassion flows over the top of your head and forehead, just like pouring honey slowly over your head.
- Let yourself experience the ease as the compassion flows over your face.
- Take a deep breath and rest in the knowledge that this light is available for you all the time. Connecting to light or a sense of universal compassion is a bigger picture intervention for you.
- Talk about the experience of engaging in this exercise. How helpful was it?

In this lesson, coping skills, bigger picture skills, mindfulness, acceptance, self-compassion, and improve the moment were all covered. You were also asked to check in regarding your intention. You are prepared to track your own progress through **Logs for Daily Living**.

Client Activity

Logs for Daily Living

Day: (Circle which day) S M T W R F S	Name:	Date:

Difficult emotions or thoughts today
(Please check)

		Please describe:
___ Anger	___ Negative thoughts about the past	
___ Sadness	___ Negative thoughts or judgments	
___ Depression	___ Worry or obsessive thoughts	
___ Anxiety	about the future	
___ Mania	___ Racing thoughts	
___ Shame	___ Difficult hallucinations	
___ Insecurity		
___ Other (emotions/thoughts): _____		

Did you use Wise Mind at all today? (Circle One)	Yes	No

I was able to *notice/observe* what was going on for me (used *mindfulness skills*) Comments:	Yes	No

I was able to *accept* my emotions/thoughts without being immediately reactive Comments:	Yes	No

I noticed that *staying aware of the breath* helped me stay more calm than usual Comments:	Yes	No

I found a way to *improve the moment* Comments (Which strategies did you use?):	Yes	No

Client Activity (*Continued*)

I connected with the *bigger picture* (deeper purpose,
higher power)   Yes   No
Comments:

I did a mindfulness practice today (3 minutes)
to strengthen my *overall skills*   Yes   No
Circle: 3-minute breathing   walking   praying   yoga
mindful   eating   other_____

Check One:
_____I approached this log with a sincere *intention* to make a difference
in my life *—Or—*
_____I more or less did this log with a skeptical "*whatever*" kind
of attitude

I was able to experience *compassion for myself* today   Yes   No
(no matter how I did the log, how effectively
I addressed my emotions . . .)
Comments:

Lesson 6: Opposite Action

[First, check in regarding client recent use of Wise Mind; then, refer to the Wise Mind figure to discuss improving the moment.]

The skill of **opposite action** moves us away from reactive responses and helps us respond from a *more* rational base. When our responses come from a mindful awareness of arising emotions as well as thoughtful reasoning, we are less likely to suffer. Balancing the rational part of our mind with the emotional part of our mind is another way of being in Wise Mind.

Opposite action says breaks our common patterns of reacting to the world. Sometimes we feel anxious and our reaction is to isolate or avoid people.

Opposite action says $\Longrightarrow$ **Reach out to people**

Sometimes we feel depressed or in despair and our reaction is to not get out of bed.

Opposite action says $\Longrightarrow$ **Take some steps to get active**

Sometimes we feel angry and our reaction is tell someone off or get into an argument.

Opposite action says $\Longrightarrow$ **Be kind and try to understand him/her**
Disengage and let go

Sometimes we feel bored and our reaction is to "stir it up" or add excitement through addictive behavior (drugs/alcohol, video games, risky sex . . .)

Opposite action says $\Longrightarrow$ **Be OK with being bored**
Call a sponsor or other support person

What is a common reaction that you have when you are in the middle of difficult emotions?

_____

_____

What is an opposite action that may work for you?

_____

_____

It is important to keep in mind the following elements when using opposite action:

➤ **Mindfulness of the moment** assists you to recognize your arising emotions and your usual responses or inclinations to respond in a certain way.

➤ Sometimes just accepting the way things are and not doing anything is enough of an opposite action.

➤ Sometimes being **compassionate with yourself** is a wonderful opposite action. Instead of watching TV and beating yourself up for being lazy while you are watching, watch TV, give yourself compassion, and fully enjoy watching TV.

➤ Maybe acknowledging that you do not feel like this is a good time to use opposite action—**and feeling okay about this**—is opposite action.

➤ Sometimes taking opposite action means taking a risk. It is a risk to try new ways of dealing with the world. It is a risk to engage when you are used to staying away. It is a risk even to feel bored.

Please write/talk about how opposite action seems like a risk to you:

_____

_____

What have been some risks that you have taken that have worked out?

_____

_____

What are some risks that are not worth taking for you?

_____

_____

What are some of your doubts of using opposite action?

_____

_____

What is some way that you can practice opposite action in the next week? How strong is your **intention** to use this skill (please be honest)?

_____

_____

Sometimes opposite action can be applied when your intention is not strong. Your tendency may be "I'm not going to take that seriously, that is B S" or perhaps less strong: it's not so important that I remember to do this, just one more exercise. In this case, opposite action is just spending a few moments to **form an intention** to take this seriously. What do you think about this?

_____

_____

How much do you do work outside of sessions? Please notice your emotions and thoughts as you answer this question. This question is not meant to make you feel bad or embarrassed.

_____

_____

Client Activity

- Close your eyes or partially close your eyes. Allow your breathing to deepen and relax.
- Think of the self-critical voice that is sometimes in your life; probably everyone has this voice to one extent or another.
- Many times this voice weighs us down, and sometimes we try unhealthy escapes from this voice.
- Engage in **opposite action**—instead of having this voice hurt us or trying to ignore this voice or react to it, let it be there.
- See the voice for what it is—and tap into a voice of self-compassion. Let this voice take whatever form makes sense (connecting with the love of the universe, a higher power, the miracle of being alive . . .)
- Think of a self-compassionate action that you can engage in today, however small.

We will talk about being willing to do things and being rebellious or resistant to doing things (also called "willful"). For now, what do you think may be a reason (or reasons) that you do/do not do the outside assignments or work?

_____

_____

Here are some possibilities to consider if you are having trouble finding reasons. Do you agree or disagree with the following (adapted from Beck et al., 1993):

It's no use—nothing is going to help.   Agree   Disagree

These assignments are not worth it
to me.   Agree   Disagree

I procrastinate, then it's too late.   Agree   Disagree

I feel too disorganized to make it
happen.   Agree   Disagree

I don't like to cooperate with the
counselor.   Agree   Disagree

I don't want to have to worry about
performance.   Agree   Disagree

Lesson 7: Not Getting Stuck Doing the Usual

Interpersonal Skills and Gathering the Mind

[*First, check in regarding client recent use of Wise Mind; then refer to the Wise Mind figure to discuss improving the moment and expanding the moment.*]

Interpersonal Skills

It is helpful to deal with others and to deal with our life in a *new way*. It is difficult to do this because we are so used to falling into familiar patterns, and it sometimes seems we are stuck doing the same thing over and over again. All of us have some personal habits that cause difficulties in our relationships. We need to identify these habits and patterns so we can make some changes and have positive relationships.

If a family member, friend, or someone you lived with could be here, what would they say is positive about being with you?

_____

_____

If a family member, friend, or someone you lived with could be here, what would they say is a situation that is difficult for you and makes you unpleasant to be with? Please be honest.

_____

_____

What makes you hard to be with? In other words, what do you do (lose your temper, yell, put someone down, threaten, become intense, do not listen)?

_____

_____

Client Activity

Some people are used to blocking communication rather than trying to understand the other person or trying sincerely—without blame—to express their own needs. Do you do any of the following? (Check the column, and please be as honest as possible)

	Yes	No
Discounting other people's needs or feelings		
Withdrawing ("I am pulling back because what's the use")		
Threatening ("Do what I want or I will hurt you or yell or have a tantrum")		
Blaming others for the tension or problem you feel		
Put down ("Why do you want that all the time; that's ridiculous")		
Guilt-tripping ("If you don't trust me, something is wrong with you")		
Derailing (Get off topic or bring focus to you/not other)		
Focus on punishing the other		

Adapted from McKay, Wood, & Brantley (2007).

How much would you like to change the way you deal with important people in your life? Please explain.

_____

_____

Sometimes the way we behave with others creates suffering but at the same time we kind of like it. Not only is it familiar, but we may feel powerful getting angry or we may feel like we cannot get our needs met anyway, so "what's the use."

What reason(s) do you have that contribute to your continued behavior?

_____

_____

The **opposite action** skill that was in the prior lesson is helpful. When we find ourselves in a situation where we are *triggered* we can notice—**with our mindfulness**—what is happening. Rather than doing things the same way, we may be able to make **other choices**.

Instead of being angry and yelling, we can be kind and try to understand.

Instead of withdrawing, we can be involved.

Instead of having a tantrum and being resistant, we can calm ourselves and cooperate.

Instead of continuing the fight, we can pull out and protect ourselves.

Instead of staying vulnerable to abuse, we can take care ourselves and do our best to stay safe.

Instead of threatening, we can listen and compromise.

Instead of making it "all about us," we can try to learn about the other person's needs.

Which of these apply to you? How much are you able to make a difference in your relationship with others?

_____

_____

Acting mindfully and accepting what is happening makes time for us to not react and to thoughtfully consider the best way to interact with others. Gathering the mind is a part of this process.

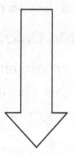

Not Getting Stuck Doing the Usual: Gathering the Mind

Gathering the mind is a vital part of mindfulness. When our mind is focused in the present moment, we experience a sense of well-being and calmness. We learn to appreciate the moment and soon learn that life is nothing more than one moment after another. We experience this when we bring our mind into the present and become fully engaged with what we are doing. If our mind is drifting away, we bring it back to the present activity. One common way to experience the richness of mindfulness is to mindfully eat a raisin (see Kabat-Zinn, 1990).

As we slow down and smell the roses (or coffee), we see the potential for mindfulness to **soothe** us in the midst of difficulty or to **connect** us to something bigger. All religious traditions introduce ritual to mindfully connect us to sacredness. We will do the exercise slowly, so please wait for each step before moving ahead. Then we will discuss what the exercise seems to mean.

➤ Look at the raisin. See what you notice and describe it. Have the description be what your eyes see and *not* be an analysis (for example, do not say, "It looks like ..." or "it is actually a dried grape").

➤ Feel the raisin. Describe what you feel without judgment.

➤ Put the raisin in your mouth without chewing it. What is your experience?

➤ Chew the raisin slowly. Chew it 10 or more times, but do not swallow it. What do you notice?

➤ Swallow the raisin. Describe your experience.

➤ You may have a commentary on the experience—notice that these are thoughts about the experience. What has it been like to gather your mind in this way?

What *mindfulness experience(s)* (3-minute breathing exercise, mindful eating, mindful listening) will you commit to between now and the next time we meet?

_____

_____

What *opposite action* will you undertake that has to do with interpersonal skills?

_____

_____

What will *increase the likelihood* that you will complete the commitment?

_____

_____

If you can, let go of the fear or resistance that goes along with making the commitment. *You will be welcomed back and completely accepted whether you complete your commitment or not.*

Exercise 8: Friend to Self: Willing Participation and Mindful Walking

[First, check in regarding client recent use of Wise Mind; then, refer to the Wise Mind figure to discuss improving the moment and expanding the moment.]

Change
Change proclaims its
dominance. "Just try
and stay the same,"
it taunts. "See how
long the status quo
will last before it's
blasted into newness
by the now."

Change isn't always
Flashy like the Grand
Canyon. Sometimes
it's subtle, like the
blinking of an eyelash
or the floating of a
feather on the wind.

Say yes, and change
will take you somewhere
unexpected. Say no,
and you'll end up in
the same place,
resisting all the while.

I'd rather go willingly
and see if the journey
itself just might be
worth the ride.

Danna Faulds
(Reprinted with permission; may be photo-
copied as part of practitioner's lessons.)

When we learn to engage deeply with mindfulness in the present moment, we gain appreciation for the world as it is. We also do things more effectively and we reduce our fight-or-flight response for various activities.

Willingness Versus Willfulness

We are able to engage with life in the moment when we "go willingly," as it says in the poem. When we are willing, we are open to trying new things, we approach situations with a positive attitude, and we may be willing to grow.

However, many times our reactive, reptilian mind puts out an immediate "**no**," which serves to prevent us from being present in an open-hearted way. We also may be stuck in the same place with our resistant no, as suggested in the poem.

What are the ways that you are *willful* in your life—you decline to participate? (Some people have translated willful as WTF—no way!, in other words, the opposite of *willing*.)

_____

_____

How does your willfulness close you off to new ways of living life or new information?

_____

_____

How much does willfulness keep you feeling safe?

_____

_____

How much have you been willful while in counseling?

_____

_____

Willingness is about being open to engaging in new ways, making some changes, or being open to new ideas.

Client Activity

Make a tight fist. Imagine you are holding on to something—your way of thinking and doing things. You do not want to let go. That is *willfulness.*

Now slowly open your fingers. Let the air flow over and around your hand. You may sense that you are letting go. If a bird were in your hand, it would have flown away. Open both hands and let your palms face the air. That is *willingness.*

What are the advantages and disadvantages of *willfulness?*

_____

_____

What are the advantages and disadvantages of *willingness?*

_____

_____

Exercise

We will do some mindful walking for a few minutes. There will be no right or wrong way to walk, but I will give you a few guidelines. I ask you to consider adopting a willing approach to the exercise.

Let's discuss the part of you that does not want to do this activity. What is the reactive mind saying (the mind that is willful/does not want to "go along with the program")?

What is the part of you that is willing? What does this part say? Assume the willing, Wise Mind and speak from this perspective.

Mindful Walking

Marsha Linehan discusses three possibilities for walking. One person is walking toward a stage and is about to receive an award relating to outstanding achievement; another is walking to the bathroom; and another is walking from a jail cell to the guillotine because he is about to have his head chopped off. In essence, all three people are just walking. That is the spirit of walking that we will engage in. Notice your feet touching the ground and notice your breath. Place gentle attention on each element. As thoughts pass or you are drawn to sense objects, notice the thoughts or what you are drawn to and continue to walk slowly.

➢ You may be assisted in your mindful walking efforts with the words *lift, step, place.* You notice as you stride that your back foot *lifts* from the ground, that your foot moves in the air to *step* forward, then the foot *places* itself on the ground.

The language is focused on how the foot moves—it is not about what "you" do to the foot. Be with the foot—lift, step, place.

Remember that there is no right or wrong way to do this exercise. Notice the judgments that you have about yourself, about the leader or the exercise, and see if you can return to your walking and breath. Develop a gentle approach if your mind happens to drift (and it will)!

Have **compassion for yourself** as you do this exercise.

What was your experience doing this exercise?

_____

_____

How much did you willfully participate?

_____

_____

What are the reasons that we do not often walk with this kind of mindfulness?

_____

_____

How valuable do you think this exercise was for you?

_____

_____

Notice that your opinions about the exercise are "stories" about the exercise. These stories are where we spend a lot of time judging and commenting.

We can regulate our emotions better if we can see when we are telling stories about things.

When we can tell the difference between

---

walking

vs.

walking + our story about walking

---

we will be more in Wise Mind and be less reactive.

What mindful practice will you engage in over this week? How willing are you to make this commitment?

_____

_____

Lesson 9: Primary and Secondary Emotions

[*First, check in regarding client recent use of Wise Mind; then, refer to the Wise Mind figure to discuss improving the moment and expanding the moment.*]

Review of Emotion Regulation

When we are able to *recognize* and be mindful of our emotions, *then our emotions* **do not** *control us to quite the same degree.* We can see emotions for what they are—temporary feeling states—rather than having the sense that our emotional state is all there is in the world. **When we become proficient at mindfully experiencing our emotions, we become less reactive and less knocked off center**. We learn to ride the waves of our emotional life and experience that we are more effective in our relationships and that we are more at peace. In this manner, our Wise Mind takes care of our emotional life.

Overall Strategies for Emotion Regulation

➤ Increase mindfulness to current emotions; this prevents extensive lapses into secondary emotions and story building (see below).

➤ Identify functions of emotions (e.g., fight–freeze–flight) or as attempt to control others.

➤ Reduce vulnerability to "emotion mind." Engage in activities that increase a sense of competence and living a balanced, healthy life.

➤ Increase positive emotional events.

➤ Take opposite action—do something nice for a person you are angry at, approach something you fear, relax when feeling constricted.

Primary and Secondary Emotions As we enhance our awareness regarding our emotional life, we find that some emotions that seem naturally expressed and appear to arise almost automatically are actually secondary to emotions that may be more vulnerable for us. It is important to identify our primary—*truest*—emotion. We are sometimes running from experiencing the primary emotion, and we are often not aware that we are doing this!! When we run like this, it is hard to express our authentic selves, we become more unregulated, and it is hard for people to get close to us.

> When you allow
> the moment to
> offer up its perfect
> response, what is
> the free and true
> experience of you?
>
> Danna Faulds
> (Excerpted from *Burn the Rope*.
> Reprinted with permission; may be photo-
> copied as part of practitioner's lessons.)

Features of Primary and Secondary Emotions

➤ "Secondary emotions are complicated, nonadaptive patterns of emotions *about* emotions" (Spradlin, 2002).

➤ Identifying secondary emotions helps us to understand our truest feelings, be more accepting of our inner world, and be more effective interpersonally.

➤ Some of us move quickly to secondary emotions, and we may become lost in a sea of emotions.

➤ Mindfulness of our emotions is useful in order to slow down the process, tune into body sensations, and identify what our true, primary emotion is.

Client Activity

Despair about sadness/disappointment

Anger about sadness/hurt

Shame for being embarrassed

⟹ Describe each for *you & think of* an example

Self-loathing for being sad

Guilty about being contented

Anxiety about joy ending/grief

Anger about being overwhelmed

Shame about anger

Which one of these is the most important to keep in mind when you are with people?

Please mention why it is the most important.

_____

_____

_____

_____

Lesson 10: Friend to Self: Doing What Is Needed and Self-Care

When we see clearly and mindfully, we notice what requires our attention and then we become aware of our response. We use our Wise Mind to:

1. Clearly see that we have choices as we interact in the environment

2. Observe and accept our thoughts and feelings about what is presented to us

3. Choose a skillful response—*improve the moment.*

Client Activity

Imagine walking into your room and seeing a pile of garbage in plain view.

What kinds of *choices* do we have about this situation?

_____

_____

What may be some emotions or thoughts that would arise in response to seeing the pile of garbage?

_____

_____

——— Client Activity (*Continued*) ———

How much do we lean in the direction of denial or tuning out (a universal response)?

_____

_____

What are some of the benefits of denial?—AND—What are the benefits of stepping up and doing what the moment requires?

_____

_____

How much do you use WISE MIND and *step up* to do what is needed?

In general, how much do you suffer because of putting things off (procrastinating)?

_____

_____

How much do you use Wise Mind and *step up* to do what is needed?

_____

_____

Client Activity

Sometimes the mind is hijacked by powerful emotions. Our life seems to be about suffering and difficulties and little else. We can follow these steps to get relief:

- Take some breaths and be mindful of difficult emotions and thoughts.
- Accept that these emotions and thoughts are arising and notice as they become less intense.

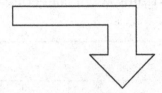

Meditation Exercise

- Take a 3-minute meditation. Allow things to move through you and focus on noticing *any degree of hope or contentment* that passes through.
- During the last minute of the breathing space, make a commitment to take care of yourself.
- Decide on some direction for *taking care of yourself*—such as calling people more, cleaning your living area, thinking more hopefully, dealing with a financial situation.

What *taking care of yourself* area did you think about?

_____

_____

How can you deal with this area in a way that feels lighthearted and *not such a burden?*

_____

_____

Many people say that they know that getting enough sleep is important for being in a good mood and for personal wellness, but it is challenging to do this. Some people do not sleep regular hours because they may try to "*cheat*" sleep – in other words, tell themselves that sleep is not important. They may stay up late hours to be on Facebook or to play video games, or they may have trouble falling asleep.

How much are you "doing what is needed" as far as sleep goes?

_____

_____

What would you like to be doing differently to take care of sleep?

_____

_____

If you are having trouble falling asleep or staying asleep, you can apply the same mindfulness and acceptance skills to sleep as you do to the rest of your life.

➤ Take things one moment at a time. *Let go of stories* about how long you have been awake and let go of questions like, "When am I ever going to fall (back) asleep?" You are awake in this one moment; that is all you have to notice.

➤ Mindfully relax different parts of your body. As you exhale, you may release tension in your head, then your forehead, then your cheekbones and jaw, then your neck. . . . Take it slowly and remember there is no "doing it right or wrong." If you make it through your entire body, do it again. You are serving your body well, even if you are not sleeping.

➤ Remember, getting frustrated or angry about sleeping will not help you get to sleep. As much as you can, notice, accept, then let go of your reactivity about staying awake.

Other suggestions for sleep are offered by Miklowitz (2011):

➤ Do not let stress enter the bedroom, such as arguments, e-mail, or texts.

➤ "Give yourself time to unwind before sleep" (p. 174). A ritual like tea drinking may be helpful.

➤ Do not get competitive with yourself about sleep time.

➤ Listen to a relaxation tape.

➤ Do not watch violent movies or television before bedtime.

➤ Maintain a fairly regular bedtime.

➤ Get up at a similar time each day.

➤ Reduce or eliminate drug/alcohol use.

➤ Speak to a medical provider about possible medication.

➤ Do not eat a lot before bed.

Sleeping well may be quite challenging, particularly if you have bipolar disorder, deal with depression, or have a substance use history. Sometimes you may be angry and frustrated enough that you feel like it's no use, and you do not try to make changes to your sleep routine or your attitude about sleep.

What information has been helpful for you to help you deal with your sleep situation?

_____

_____

Remember to maintain a compassionate approach with yourself as you deal with these issues.

Lesson 11: Getting Grounded: Finding Wellness Amidst Distress, Anxiety, and Worry

Grounding helps bring your focus *away* from emotional pain. If you are overwhelmed with emotions or feeling numb, grounding helps you find the middle point. Grounding is different than what has been taught so far: *mindfully noticing* and *accepting* what is going on internally—your thoughts and emotions. Instead of being intimate with your internal life,

> *"Grounding puts healthy distance between you and negative feelings."*

(Najavits, 2002, p. 133)

We will focus on a physically oriented way of grounding ourselves. Here are the principles:

➤ You can decide to use grounding as soon as you start feeling highly anxious, distressed, or overwhelmed.

➤ Scan your surroundings. Notice the room or the sunlight. Notice your feet on the ground and perhaps your hands touching a chair.

➤ Stay in the present. Do not dredge up thoughts about the past or indulge in worries about the future.

➤ Notice your body. As you make movements, notice your hands in your lap, your thighs on a chair, and so on.

➤ Notice your breath. You may recite a word as you inhale and exhale. For example, as you inhale: "safe"; as you exhale: "mountain."

➤ You may add a coping statement for yourself: For example, "I will be okay."

─────── **Client Activity** ───────

Engage in a grounding exercise. Bring the *intention* that you will get something out of it, as well as a willingness to experiment and grow. Have someone read the steps above to you and remember the emphasis is on reducing the emotional charge and feeling okay *right now,* not on fixing the problem.

How much does the grounding exercise help you get a healthy distance from distress or anxiety?

_____

_____

What part of this exercise is the most important for you (slowing the breath, noticing your body's contact with something, having a phrase that is soothing or an image that is positive)?

_____

_____

What would help you to remember to use grounding?

_____

_____

When is the *most likely time* that it would make sense to use grounding (the kinds of times where grounding would help you the most)?

_____

_____

_____

Assignment Suggestion: Attempt a grounding exercise before the next session. Notice how helpful it was to you.

Worrying and Letting Go of Worry

Worry is an emotion that primarily comes from our stories about what may happen in the future. The intensity of our worry lessens when we can see how it arises and we can let go of the thoughts that fuel it.

Discuss the things that you worry about and talk about how often you worry. Worry is a part of *ruminative thought* that contributes to depression and anxiety. It is important to be aware that when we are worrying, we are engaging in a particular activity that we can choose to let go of. Letting go of worry is a gift.

Client Activity

- Imagine that you are worrying about something.
- Apply mindfulness and notice that this mental activity is called worrying.
- See how you are generating stories about the future—you are leaving this moment.
- Make a commitment to *not fuse with worry.*
- *Fusing* means that you are so strongly connected to a mental or emotional process that it feels like your *entire life is this experience!*
- Take some breaths and make a choice to engage in another activity (something other than worrying).

Interpersonal Skills and Worry

Worry can also interfere with how we interact with other people. If you anticipate that people will not like you or that you are going to "look stupid," it will be hard to feel comfortable being with others. Sometimes you may project your own negative thinking about yourself onto others. For example, "She probably thinks that I'm not worth hanging around." This may be a thought that you have about yourself and you are projecting this thought on another person.

Client Activity

How do you handle worries when you are involved with other people?

_____

_____

_____

What kinds of worries do you have that take a lot of energy (concerns about what others think about you, worries about your children, worries about your partner)?

_____

_____

It is okay to have worries, the question is what is the *best way to address them*?

Does thinking about the same worries over and over help?

_____

How may the serenity prayer help you with some of your worries (see next page)?

_____

_____

The Serenity Prayer
God, grant me the serenity
To accept the things I cannot change
The courage to change the things I can
And the wisdom to know the difference.

The emphasis in using our Wise Mind is to stay in the present. Sometimes, though, our worries alert us to concerns regarding *not being safe*, or that we are about to engage in *risky action*. The serenity prayer provides direction about what to do with these worries.

Although the emotional charge from worry may alert us, especially in terms of fight-or-flight, we eventually want to lower the charge because it is exhausting, it is overwhelming, and it does not help us.

Worry tends to build on itself to the point where our overall anxiety takes over.

Use mindfulness to see worry for what it is—negative thoughts fueling emotion which is fueling more negative thoughts.

Decide on moving in the direction of *accepting and letting go* or *making a change.*

Be *compassionate with yourself*. Sometimes making a change does not mean doing something dramatic; it may mean taking one step like speaking to a counselor about something or telling yourself the truth about feeling vulnerable.

Client Activity

How do you want to handle the big worries in your life?

_____

_____

_____

What are your overall strategies for *improving the moment* as the worries arise?

_____

_____

What are some longer term strategies concerning some of your worries?

_____

_____

How much will you connect with spirituality or the *bigger picture* to deal with worries?

_____

_____

What role does *self-compassion* play in dealing with worries?

_____

_____

Lesson 12: Finding the Zone: Moving From Suffering to Balance

It is helpful if you can find the zone where you are able to meet life and feel balanced. Elaine Miller-Karas and Laurie Leitch (2009) call this the *resilient zone*. In this zone, you feel like you can take care of yourself. If there are stressors, they seem manageable. Your nervous system is actually in balance *even in the middle of difficulties.*

When you are not in the resilient zone, you are stressed and do not feel balanced. You are stuck in either hyperarousal, which means stuck on high, or you are in hypoarousal, which means stuck on low. It looks like this:

High   Hyperactivity / Hypervigilance / Mania / Anxiety / Panic / Rage / Pain

---

RESILIENT ZONE: Maintain healthy functioning / have positive emotions

---

Low   Depression / Disconnection / Exhaustion / Fatigue / Numbness / Boredom

Adapted from Miller-Karas & Leitch (2009).

Many times when we are stressed, we try to "think our way out" of situations. As we do this, we may become more and more stressed and can move out of our resilient zone.

Strategies for Returning to the Resilient Zone

Keep tuning into how you are doing emotionally. Be mindful/ slow down and accept what and how you are feeling.

Step back from the intensity.

Don't focus on solving the problem.

Don't keep repeating the same information or going over the same details over and over.

Ask the questions:

How can I take care of myself now, in this present moment?

How can I change from suffering and being triggered to feeling more balanced?

Allow yourself to "chill." Make a joke or have coffee with someone. You don't do your best processing or problem solving when you are activated. This advice is not about denial or minimizing your suffering but about not being highly triggered and unbalanced. This is called pendulating. Move like the pendulum *from high stress to wellness*.

Client Activity

When you move out of the resilient zone do you tend to go high or low?

_____

_____

What happens in your body to let you know that you are getting triggered?

_____

_____

Your commitment to stay in the resilient zone is an act of *self-compassion*.

Client Activity

Approach this activity with a sense of *willingness* and the *intention* that you will get something out of it. The goal is to be able to tap into something or connect with someone supportive that *comforts* us.

- Let yourself close your eyes or partially close your eyes.
- If that is too stressful—you can keep your eyes open and notice your feet on the ground and your hands on the chair.
- Let your breathing slow down and see what it is like to witness your breath.
- Imagine a state of wellness where something or someone is *comforting you*—making you feel okay about life in this moment.
- Imagine that you can call on this person or resource at different times and that you will feel comforted even when things are difficult.
- You deserve to have this *comforting source* in your life.

How much will you be able to rely on this comfort in your life?

_____

_____

What would stop you from connecting with comfort (getting into the resilient zone) when you are in distress, despair, or rage?

_____

_____

Taking care of yourself in this way is an act of self-compassion— How much compassion do you have for yourself?

_____

_____

What would having more compassion for yourself look like?

_____

_____

Daffodils
A hundred daffodils
lift their faces
to the sun,
never noticing
their own golden light.

Danna Faulds
(Reprinted with permission; may be photo-
copied as part of practitioner's lessons.)

What does this poem mean to you?

_____

_____

What about your own golden light?

_____

_____

Write about being compassionate with yourself. Experiment with trying to be compassionate. How much do you deserve this kind of compassion? How much would it make a difference in your life?

Lesson 13: Self-Nurturance and Joy

It is important to sort out what activities we can engage in to take care of ourselves and that bring us self-nurturance and joy. Sometimes we are confused about nurturing ourselves because of the following reasons:

> ➤ We may not have been nurtured consistently while growing up, so now it is hard to know what it is like to nurture ourselves.

> ➤ We have become used to experiencing pain and perhaps we have identified as being a victim, which means that we believe that we are not supposed to feel good.

> ➤ We have sought patterns of behavior or addiction that bring some relief but also bring painful consequences.

> ➤ We have been taught that there is not much pleasure to get out of life—this lesson can come from being around negative, abusive, or unhappy people.

What may be part of the reason it is hard for you to self-nurture (taking care of yourself and living joyfully)?

_____

_____

There are ways to build self-nurturing into your life:

Have the intention to experience joy—Recognize that experiencing joy is part of your birthright.

Find meaning in difficulty—This **expand the moment**, bigger picture approach helps you deal with hard times. You can accept the difficult times and doing so sets the stage for seeing into how your courage has lifted you to the place you are today. Albert Einstein said, "In the middle of difficulty lies opportunity."

Focus on moment-to-moment self-nurturing and joy—Ask the question: "How can I take care of myself now?"

Build a list of activities that are self-nurturing—Some may be small and easily accessible (e.g., cook a meal and eat by a lit candle rather than eat fast food, meditate or pray, sit with your pet, look at a child's eyes and be truly present rather than think about what else you could be doing, do light stretching, take a bath). Some activities may be once-in-a-while (e.g., plan a celebration, go on a trip).

How much intention do you have to nurture yourself?

_____

_____

What are ways that you nurture yourself now?

_____

_____

What other ways can you add to the list?

_____

_____

As you are thinking of ways to nurture yourself, what emotions and thoughts are coming up for you—*RIGHT NOW?* (Thoughts of: *this is helpful, this is stupid, I don't like this* . . . or emotions of *guilt, fear about doing something unfamiliar, excitement, numbness . . .*)

_____

_____

Imagine that you could parent the *part of yourself* that is little, needs nurturance, and is hopeful about enjoying life.

What would you say to that little, hopeful child that is inside of you?

Please write down your honest thoughts:

_____

_____

Client Activity

Freely write down thoughts in this space about self-nurturance:

What are the practical obstacles that you have for self-nurturing?

_____

_____

How much does *self-compassion* relate to self-nurturing? How can you give yourself permission to self-nurture?

_____

_____

Mindfulness practice is actually a self-nurturing practice. You become more able to appreciate life on its own terms and—like eating the raisin—feel connected to the smallest of acts. How much will you sustain mindfulness practices?

_____

_____

Lesson 14: Effective Speech and Telling the Truth

We seek to be genuine in our relationships with people so we let others know about how we are honestly feeling or what we are honestly thinking. This level of truth telling is helpful because being clear about ourselves may help us:

Get our needs met and
Maintain healthy boundaries

We balance our truth telling with a few considerations:

Am I expressing thoughts and emotions in a way that another person can hear them or am I trying to overpower the person with how right I am and how wrong he or she is?

What is my *intention?* Am I expressing thoughts and emotions in a way to be *beneficial (helpful)* to the other person or our relationship, or am I so mad or frustrated that I am not really thinking about how helpful my words are?

How much will my words be *hurtful* to the other person? Many times we are trying to figure out whether we should say something because our words may be true and may be beneficial, but they may be hurtful. Other combinations are also possible. These considerations—*truthful, beneficial, not hurtful*—comprise the components of "right speech" in the Buddhist tradition.

Many times only one or two components of right speech are present, and sometimes we are not sure if something would be beneficial or hurtful. It is not always clear what to say to someone. Our interpersonal relationships are going to be better if the following happens:

➢ **We are clear about our intentions when we are talking.**

➢ We maintain mindful speech—that is, we do not "strike back" (fight) or avoid (flight) or go numb (freeze) because of reactivity. We notice our arising emotions and our reactive tendencies, and we *engage if it is safe to do so.*

➢ We maintain awareness of the experience of the other person *and* realize that we are not completely responsible for satisfying that person's needs.

➢ We understand that taking care of ourselves means that we will choose healthy boundaries.

Client Activity

Think of a time when you engaged in a conversation or argument that was not so skillful. How could you have relied more on Wise Mind and stated your needs in a way that would have been more effective, and perhaps:

Would have promoted dialog

Would have been more uplifting (*beneficial*) for the both of you

Would have involved more *truth telling* about your vulnerabilities

Would have been *less hurtful* or mean spirited

What incident are you thinking about?

_____

_____

What could you have done differently?

_____

_____

Mud of the Moment
Truth lives in the mud
of this moment. It exists
in the messy interplay of
emotions and relationship,
in the personality traits
I'd rather leave behind.

> To experience truth
> doesn't take sainthood,
> or dissolving my desires.
> It requires diving into
> the muck and mire of
> what's here, feeling
> the anxiety or fear,
> knowing the entirety
> of me without hiding
> from the shadows or
> from light.
>
> The lotus never
> blooms without
> sinking roots in the mud.
>
> Danna Faulds
> (Reprinted with permission; may be photo-
> copied as part of practitioner's lessons.)

The Truth and Wise Mind Practices

Mindfulness helps us to see the truth of the present moment. Acceptance is about coming face-to-face with reality exactly as it is. These are practices that shine the light on truth even when—as the poem says—"the truth lies in the mud of the moment."

The truth holds power in the 12-step tradition. In the fourth step, you come to terms with who you are, where you've been, what your struggles are. In the Christian church, the slogan "the truth will set you free" is often repeated.

As you head toward wellness and recovery, what is the role of *the truth* in your life?

_____

_____

How much can you relate to the idea that the roots of the lotus are found in the mud? In other words, the roots of your beauty are in the fertile soil of your difficult experiences and challenging life.

_____

_____

How can you maintain compassion for yourself, as you become more aware of the truth?

_____

_____

Client Activity

- Take a few deep breaths.
- Continue to focus on breath or, if preferred, a repeated phrase such as "may I be safe and well."
- As you continue to settle, please listen to these words:
  You have been on a journey of truth that is quite rich. Although there is mud, your life is beautiful. See if you can appreciate the beauty of your life! See if you can appreciate the beauty of you being you.
- After 30 seconds, you can gently open your eyes fully.

What was your experience of this exercise?

_____

_____

_____

Over this next week, please keep track of times where you were mindful of what was happening for you, and you told the truth to yourself.

Lesson 15: Inspiring the World With Our Courage and Path

I've fallen in love
with my own life
in all its gloriously
messy imperfection

Danna Faulds
(Reprinted with permission; may be photo-
copied as part of practitioner's lessons.)

Your Courageous and Inspiring Life

You have developed some amazing capacities to fight through difficult times and to be at the point that you are at in life. One aspect of mindfulness involves shining the light on your thoughts and emotions that involve feeling gratified, peaceful, proud, or connected. When you think about what you have accomplished and how brave you have been, you:

Realize that you are more courageous than you have imagined;

Understand that your struggles provide lessons and inspiration for others;

Connect to your higher power or to something bigger than your day-to-day worries.

Courage

You have had difficult times in your life that you have had to overcome—simply to be sitting here today.

What kind of courage have you had in order to keep going?

There might be some "yeah but" going on. These are the messages that interfere with experiencing your own worthiness. Use Wise Mind to be mindful of the "yeah buts" and *allow yourself feel gratitude for the strength that you possess.* This manner of being in Wise Mind—being aware of your courage and feeling gratitude for your strength—promotes healing, resilience, contentment, and effectiveness.

Client Activity

Please discuss your courage to move forward in your life.

_____

_____

_____

(See if you can notice and let go of any "yeah but" kind of thinking and let yourself fully accept thoughts and emotions related to your personal courage.)

Inspiration for Others

You have certainly made mistakes, but as you take steps forward you have the opportunity to inspire and influence others.

Who are the people that you may inspire through your courageous work and through staying on the path of wellness and recovery?

_____

_____

It is important to see that your life is a creative painting of mistakes and courage. This painting serves the world as a source of inspiration. At times, however, despair arises and it feels like you are barely hanging on for survival; these may be the times when the "eff-its" make their appearance and you contemplate giving up or relapsing.

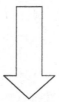

You honor your intention to use Wise Mind to mindfully notice and accept the times when "eff-it" arises, you improve the moment, and, with self-compassion, recommit to your path on behalf of your friends, your family, your community, yourself, and all the beings in the world who are counting on you.

References

Anthony, W. A. (1993). Recovery from mental illness: The guiding vision of the mental health system in the 1990's. *Innovations and Research, 2,* 17–24.

Arkowitz, H., Westra, H. A., Miller, W. R., & Rollnick, S. (2008). *Motivational interviewing in the treatment of psychological problems.* New York, NY: Guilford Press.

Beck, A. T., Wright, F. D., Newman, C. F., & Liese, B. S. (1993). *Cognitive therapy of substance abuse.* New York, NY: Guilford Press.

Bein, A. (2003). The ethnographic perspective: A new look. In J. Anderson & R. W. Carter (Eds.), *Diversity perspectives for social work practice* (pp. 133–145). Boston, MA: Pearson Education.

Bein, A. (2008). *The Zen of helping: Spiritual principles for mindful and open-hearted practice.* Hoboken, NJ: Wiley.

Bertolino, B., & Miller, S.D. (Eds.). (2012). *Manual 2: What works in therapy: A primer.* Chicago, IL: International Center for Clinical Excellence Press.

Bishop, S. R., Lau, M., Shapiro, S., Carlson, L., Anderson, N. D., Carmody, J., . . . Devins, G. (2004). Mindfulness: A proposed operational definition. *Clinical Psychology: Science and Practice, 10,* 230–241.

Blair, R. J. (2008). The amygdala and ventromedial prefrontal cortex: Functional contributions and dysfunction in psychopathy. *Philosophical Transactions of the Royal Society: Biological Sciences, 363,* 2557–2565. doi: 10:1098/rstb.2008.0027

Bowen, S., Chawla, N., & Marlatt, G. A. (2011). *Mindfulness-based relapse prevention for addictive behaviors: A clinician's guide.* New York, NY: Guilford Press.

Brave Heart, M. Y. H. (2007). The impact of historical trauma: The example of the Native community. In M. Bussey & J. B. Wise (Eds.), *Trauma transformed: An empowerment response* (pp. 175–193). New York, NY: Columbia University.

Briere, J., & Scott, C. (2006). *Principles of trauma therapy: A guide to symptoms, evaluation, and treatment.* Thousand Oaks, CA: Sage.

Burnam, M. A., & Watkins, K. E. (2006). Substance abuse with mental disorders. Specialized public systems and integrated care. *Health Affairs, 25*(3), 648–658.

Canda, E. R., Nakashima, M., & Furman, L. D. (2004). Ethical considerations about spirituality in social work: Insights from a national qualitative survey. *Families in Society, 85*(1), 27–35.

Carson, C. (Ed.). (1998). *The autobiography of Martin Luther King, Jr.* New York, NY: Warner Books.

Comtois, K. A., Koons, C. R., Kim, S. A., Manning, S. Y., Bellows, E., & Dimeff, L. A. (2007). In L. A. Dimeff & K. Koerner (Eds.), *Dialectical behavior therapy in clinical practice: Applications across disorders and settings* (pp. 37–68). New York, NY: Guilford Press.

Conrod, P. J., & Stewart, S. H. (2005). A critical look at dual-focused cognitive-behavioral treatments for co-morbid use and psychiatric disorders: Strengths, limitations and future directions. *Journal of Cognitive Psychotherapy, 19*(3), 261–284.

Davidson, L., Tondora, J., Lawless, M. S., O'Connell, M. J., & Rowe, M. (2009). *A practical guide to recovery-oriented practice: Tools for transforming mental health care.* New York, NY: Oxford University.

Deegan, P. E. (1995). *Principles of a recovery model.* Retrieved from http://www.power2u.org/downloads/MedicationMeeting Packet.pdf

Deegan, P. E. (2001). *Recovery as a journey of the heart.* Retrieved from http://aterhamtning.se/Recovery%20As%20a%20Journey %20of%20the%20heart.pdf

Denning, P., & Little, J. (2012). *Practicing harm reduction psycho-therapy: An alternative approach to addictions* (2nd ed.). New York, NY: Guilford Press.

DiClemente, C. C. (2006). *Addiction and change: How addictions develop and addicted people recover.* New York, NY: Guilford Press.

Dimeff, L. A., & Koerner, K. (Eds.). (2007). *Dialectical behavior therapy in clinical practice: Applications across disorders and set-tings.* New York, NY: Guilford.

Dimidjian, S., & Linehan, M. M. (2003). Mindfulness practice. In W. O'Donohue, J. E. Fisher, & S. C. Hayes (Eds.), *Cognitive behavior therapy* (pp. 229–237). Hoboken, NJ: Wiley.

Drake, R. E., Mueser, K. T., Brunette, M. F., & McHugo, G. J. (2004). A review of treatments for people with severe mental ill-nesses and co-occurring substance use disorders. *Psychiatric Rehabilitation Journal, 27*(4), 360–374. doi: 10.2975/27.2004 .360.374

Duncan, B. L., & Miller, S. D. (2000). The client's theory of change: Consulting the client in the integrative process. *Journal of Psychotherapy Integration, 10*(2), 169–187.

Duncan, B. L., Miller, S. D., & Sparks, J. A. (2004). *The heroic client: A revolutionary way to improve effectiveness through client-centered, outcome-informed therapy.* San Francisco, CA: Jossey-Bass.

Duncan, B. L., Miller, S. D., Wampold, B. E., & Hubble, M. A. (2010). *The heart and soul of change: Delivering what works in therapy* (2nd ed.). Washington, DC: American Psychological Association.

Frese, F. J. (2013, February 21). National Alliance on Mental Illness annual Pat Williams mental health dinner. Veterans Memorial Center, Davis, CA.

Frese, F. J., Stanley, J., Kress, K., & Vogel-Scibilia, S. (2001). Integrating evidence-based practices and the recovery model. *Psychiatric Services, 52*(11), 1462–1468.

Fruzetti, A. E., Iverson, K. M. (2004). Mindfulness, acceptance, validation, and "individual" psychopathology in couples. In S. C. Hayes, V. M. Follette, & M. M. Linehan (Eds.), *Mindfulness and acceptance: Expanding the cognitive-behavioral tradition* (pp.168–191). New York, NY: Guilford Press.

Fulton, P. R. (2005). Mindfulness as clinical training. In C. K. Germer, R. D. Siegel, & P. R. Fulton (Eds.), *Mindfulness and psychotherapy* (pp. 55–72). New York, NY: Guilford Press.

Gehring, W. J., & Fencsik, D. E. (2001). Functions of the medial frontal cortex in the processing of conflict and errors. *Journal of Neuroscience, 21*(23), 9430–9437. Retrieved from http://www.jneurosci.org/content/21/23/9430.full.pdf

Goleman, D. (1995). *Emotional intelligence: Why it can matter more than IQ.* New York, NY: Bantam Books.

Goleman, D. (2004). *Destructive emotions: A scientific dialog with the Dalai Lama.* New York, NY: Bantam.

Gross, J. J., & John, O. P. (2003). Individual differences in two emotion-regulation processes: Implications for affect, relationships, and well-being. *Journal of Personality and Social Psychology, 85,* 348–362.

Gross, J. J., & Thompson, R. (2007). Emotion regulation: Conceptual foundations. In J. J. Gross (Ed.), *Handbook of emotion regulation* (pp. 3–21). New York, NY: Guilford Press.

Halifax, J. (2008). Foreword. In A. Bein (Ed.), *The Zen of helping: Spiritual principles for mindful and open-hearted practice* (pp. xiii–xiv). Hoboken, NJ: Wiley.

Hayes, S. C., & Lillis, J. (2012). *Acceptance and commitment therapy: Theories of psychotherapy.* Washington, DC: American Psychological Association.

Herman, J. (1997). *Trauma and recovery: The aftermath of violence—from domestic abuse to political terror.* New York, NY: Basic Books.

Herman, J. L., Perry, J., & Van der Kolk, B. A. (1989). Childhood trauma in borderline personality disorder. *American Journal of Psychiatry, 146*(4), 490–495.

Hewitt, J., & Coffey, M. (2005). Therapeutic working relationships with people with schizophrenia: Literature review. *Journal of Advanced Nursing, 52*(5), 561–570.

Hodge, D. R. (2005). Spiritual ecograms: A new assessment instrument for identifying clients' strengths in space and across time. *Families in Society, 86*(2), 287–296.

Ina, S. (1999). *Children of the camps* [Video]. Mill Valley, CA: Psychotherapy.net.

Kabat-Zinn, J. (1990). *Full catastrophe living: Using the wisdom of your body and mind to face stress, pain, and illness.* New York, NY: Dell.

Koerner, K. (2012). *Doing dialectical behavior therapy: A practical guide.* New York, NY: Guilford Press.

Koole, S. (2009). The psychology of emotion regulation: An integrative review. *Cognition & Emotion, 23*(1), 4–41. doi: 10.1080/02699930802619031

Linehan, M. (1993). *Skills training manual for treating borderline personality disorder.* New York, NY: Guilford Press.

Linehan, M., (2005). *This one moment: Skills for everyday mindfulness* [Video]. Seattle, WA: Behavioral Tech.

Littell, J. H. (2010). Evidence-based practice: Evidence or orthodoxy? In B. L. Duncan, S. D. Miller, B. E. Wampold, & M. A. Hubble (Eds.), *The heart and soul of change: Delivering what works in therapy* (2nd ed., pp. 167–198). Washington, DC: American Psychological Association.

Luoma, J. B., Hayes, S. C., & Walter, R. D. (2007). *Learning ACT: An acceptance and commitment therapy skills-training manual for therapists.* Oakland, CA: New Harbinger.

Malekoff, A. (2004). *Group work with adolescents: Principles and practice* (2nd ed.). New York, NY: Guilford Press.

Marra, T. (2004). *Depressed & anxious: The dialectical behavior therapy workbook for overcoming depression & anxiety.* Oakland, CA: New Harbinger.

Mauss, I., Levenson, R., McCarter, L., Wilhelm, F., & Gross, J. (2005). The tie that binds? Coherence among emotion, experience, behavior and physiology. *Emotion, 5,* 175–190.

McKay, M., Wood, J. C., & Brantley, J. (2007). *The dialectical behavior therapy skills workbook: Practical DBT exercises for learning mindfulness, interpersonal effectiveness, emotion regulation & distress tolerance.* Oakland. CA: New Harbinger.

McMain, S., Sayrs, J. H., Dimeff, L. A., & Linehan, M. M. (2007). Dialectical behavior therapy for individuals with borderline personality disorder and substance dependence. In L. A. Dimeff & K. Koerner (Eds.), *Dialectical behavior therapy in clinical practice: Applications across disorders and settings* (pp. 145–173). New York, NY: Guilford Press.

Miklowitz, D. J. (2011). *The bipolar survival guide: What you and your family need to know* (2nd ed.). New York, NY: Guilford Press.

Miller-Karas, E., & Leitch, L. (2009). *Trauma resiliency model: Healing one step at a time.* Claremont, CA: Trauma Resource Institute.

Minkoff, K., & Cline, C. A. (2006). Dual diagnosis capability: Moving from concept to implementation. *Journal of Dual Diagnosis, 2*(2), 121–134.

Mollica, R. F. (2006). *Healing invisible wounds: Paths to hope and recovery in a violent world.* Orlando, FL: Harcourt Books.

Najavits, L. M. (2002). *Seeking safety: A treatment manual for PTSD and substance abuse.* New York, NY: Guilford Press.

National Alliance on Mental Illness. (2003). *Dual diagnosis and integrated treatment of mental illness and substance abuse disorder.* Retrieved from http://www.nami.org/Template.cfm?Section=By_Illness&Template=/TaggedPage/TaggedPageDisplay.cfm&TPLID=54&ContentID=23049

Neff, K. (2011). *Self-compassion: Stop beating yourself up and leave insecurity behind.* New York, NY: HarperCollins.

New York Times Video. (2011). *Health: The power of rescuing others.* Retrieved from http://www.nytimes.com/video/2011/06/23/health/100000000877082/the-power-of-rescuing-others .html#100000000877082

Nhat Hanh, T. (1998). *The heart of the Buddha's teaching: Transforming suffering into peace, joy, & liberation.* Berkeley, CA: Parallax.

Norcross, J. C., & Wampold, B. E. (2011). Evidence-based therapy relationships: Research conclusions and clinical practices. *Psychotherapy, 48*(1), 98–102.

Prochaska, J. O., DiClemente, C. C., & Norcross, J. C. (1992). In search of how people change: Applications to addictive behaviors. *American Psychologist, 47,* 1102–1114.

Rapp, C., & Goscha, R. J. (2006). *The strengths model: Case management with people with psychiatric disabilities* (2nd ed.). New York, NY: Oxford University Press.

Reynolds, S. K., Wolbert, R., Abney-Cunningham, G., & Patterson, K. (2007). Dialectical behavior therapy for assertive community treatment teams. In L. A. Dimeff & K. Koerner (Eds.), *Dialectical behavior therapy in clinical practice: Applications across disorders and settings* (pp. 298–325). New York, NY: Guilford Press.

Richards, R. S., & Sehr, D. P. (2011). *The usefulness of dialectical behavior therapy in substance abuse groups* (Unpublished master's thesis). California State University, Sacramento.

Robins, C. J., Schmidt, H., & Linehan, M. M. (2004). Dialectical behavior therapy: Synthesizing radical acceptance with skillful means. In S. C. Hayes, V. M. Follett, & M. M. Linehan (Eds.), *Mindfulness and acceptance: Expanding the cognitive-behavioral tradition* (pp. 30–44). New York, NY: Guilford Press.

Saleebey, D. (2012). *The strengths perspective in social work practice* (6th ed.). New York, NY: Pearson.

Schutte, N., Manes, R., & Malouff, J. (2009). Antecedent-focused emotion regulation, response modulation and well-being. *Current Psychology, 28*(1), 21–31. doi: 10.1007/s12144-009-9004-3

Segal, Z. V., Williams, J. M., & Teasdale, J. D. (2002). *Mindfulness-based cognitive therapy for depression: A new approach for preventing relapse.* New York, NY: Guilford.

Sells, D., Rowe, M., Fisk, D., & Davidson, L. (2003). Violent victimization of persons with co-occuring psychiatric and substance abuse disorders. *Psychiatric Services, 54,* 1253–1257.

Shulman, L. (1999). *Skills of helping individuals, families, groups, and communities* (4th ed.). Beverly, MA: Wadsworth.

Siegel, D. J. (2003). An interpersonal neurobiology of psychotherapy: The developing mind and the resolution of trauma. In M. F. Solomon & D. J. Siegel (Eds.), *Healing trauma: Attachment, mind, body and brain* (pp. 1–56). New York, NY: W. W. Norton.

Siegel, D. J. (2010). *Mindsight: The new science of personal transformation.* New York, NY: Bantam.

Slade, M. (2009). *Personal recovery and mental illness: A guide for mental health professionals.* New York, NY: Cambridge University Press.

Spradlin, S. E. (2002). *Don't let your emotions run your life: How dialectical behavior therapy can put you in control.* Oakland, CA: New Harbinger.

Sterling, S., Chi, F., & Hinman, A. (2006). Integrating care for people with co-occurring alcohol and other drug, medical and mental health conditions. *Alcohol Research and Health, 33*(4), 338–349.

Strosahl, K. D., & Robinson, P. J. (2008). *The mindfulness & acceptance workbook for depression: Using acceptance & commitment therapy to move through depression & create a life worth living.* Oakland, CA: New Harbinger.

Substance Abuse and Mental Health Services Administration Blog. (2012). *SAMHSA's working definitions of recovery updated.* Retrieved from http://blog.samhsa.gov/2012/03/23definition-of-recovery-updated

Thompson, R. (2006). *Raising Cain: Exploring the inner lives of America's boys* [Video]. Arlington, VA: Public Broadcasting Service.

Trull T. J., Sher, K. J., Minks-Brown, C., Durbin, J., & Burr, R. (2000). Borderline personality disorder and substance use disorders: A review and integration. *Clinical Psychology Review*, 20(2), 235–253.

Tsai, M., Kohlenberg, R. J., Kanter, J., Kohlenberg, B., Follette, W., & Callaghan, G. (2009). *A guide to functional analytic psychotherapy: Awareness, courage, love and behaviorism*. New York, NY: Springer.

United States Department of Veterans Affairs, National Center for PTSD. (2012). *New diagnostic criteria for PTSD to be released: DSM-5*. Washington, DC: Author. Retrieved from http://www.ptsd.va.gov/professional/pages/diagnostic_criteria_dsm-5.asp.

Van der Kolk, B. A., MacFarlane, A. C, & Weisaeth, L. (Eds.), (1996). *Traumatic stress: The effects of overwhelming experience on the body, mind, and society*. New York, NY: Guilford Press.

Van Gelder, K. (2010). *The Buddha and the borderline: A memoir*. Oakland, CA: New Harbinger.

Walsh, J. (2013) *The recovery philosophy and direct social work practice*. Chicago, IL: Lyceum.

Westra, H. A., & Dozois, D. J. (2008). Integrating motivational interviewing into the treatment of anxiety. In H. Arkowitz, H. A. Westra, W. R. Miller, & S. Rollnick (Eds.), *Motivational interviewing in the treatment of psychological problems* (pp. 26–56). New York, NY: Guilford Press.

Wilson, W. G., & Smith, R. H. (1939). *Alcoholics Anonymous*. United States: Alcoholics Anonymous World Services.

Zanarini, M. C., Williams, A., Lewis, R. Reich, R., Vera, S., Marino, M., . . . Frandenburg, F. (1997). Reported pathological childhood experiences associated with the development of borderline personality disorder. *American Journal of Psychiatry*, *154*, 1101–1106.

Appendix

LOGS FOR DAILY LIVING

Day: (Circle which day) S M T W R F S	Name:	Date:

Difficult emotions or thoughts today (Please check)	
___ Anger ___ Negative thoughts about the past ___ Sadness ___ Negative thoughts or judgments ___ Depression ___ Worry or obsessive thoughts about the future ___ Anxiety ___ Mania ___ Racing thoughts ___ Shame ___ Difficult hallucinations ___ Insecurity ___ Other (emotions/thoughts): _____	*Please describe:*

Did you use Wise Mind at all today? (Circle One)	Yes	No

I was able to *notice/observe* what was going on for me (used *mindfulness skills*) Comments:	Yes	No

I was able to *accept* my emotions/thoughts without being immediately reactive Comments:	Yes	No

I noticed that *staying aware of the breath* helped me stay more calm than usual Comments:	Yes	No

I found a way to *improve the moment* Comments (Which strategies did you use?):	Yes	No

I connected with the ***bigger picture*** (deeper purpose,
higher power)   Yes   No
Comments:

I did a mindfulness practice today (3 minutes)
to strengthen my ***overall skills***   Yes   No
Circle: 3-minute breathing   walking   praying   yoga
mindful eating   other_____

Check One:
_____I approached this log with a sincere ***intention*** to make a
difference in my life *—Or—*
_____I more or less did this log with a skeptical "*whatever*" kind of
attitude

I was able to experience ***compassion for myself*** today   Yes   No
(no matter how I did the log, how effectively
I addressed my emotions . . .)
Comments:

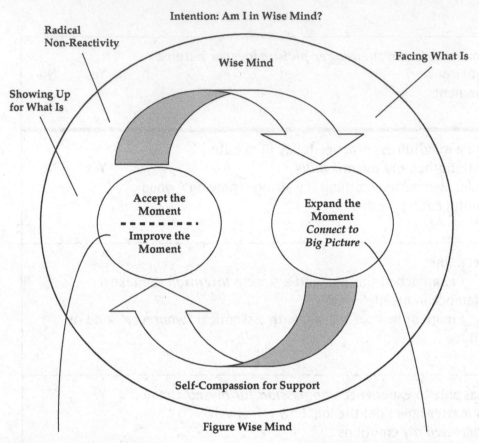

Figure Wise Mind

Being with breath & not reacting.
Letting go of judgments.
Engaging in what soothes/I enjoy.
Mindfulness—one thing at a time.
Friend to self & support from others.
Grounding self & embracing safety.
Distraction from distress.
Effective speech & interpersonal skills.
Awareness of primary & secondary emotions.
Doing what is needed & not getting hooked.

My "job" is about healing & freedom.
What does my higher power want for me?
I belong on the planet.
Life is more than this moment of suffering.
What is my deepest purpose?
Courage to tell the truth to self.

Acknowledgments

In deep appreciation of Mom and Dad, Bella, and Sam.

Emily and Mike, you shine the light on the possibilities for living with mental illness. Your courage and heart and willingness to engage, risk, and tell the truth are sources of precious inspiration.

I want to thank the people who made this book possible. Dr. Robin Kennedy at Sacramento State University, thank you for supporting me and thank you for your personal emotion regulation efforts in these challenging times. Karen Larsen, Director of Behavioral Health at Communicare, I appreciate your allowing me to conduct dual diagnosis DBT-WR groups and to be part of your incredible team for 7 years. Thank you to some amazing teachers who, in different ways, contribute to the book: Joan Halifax, Jon Kabat-Zinn, and Ed Brown.

I appreciate the financial support from Sacramento State that enabled me to write this book. I feel much gratitude for the people at John Wiley & Sons, particularly Rachel Livsey, for your skilled, dedicated, and caring involvement. Thank you, Emma Spanko, for assisting with editing. I would also would like to thank the following colleagues who reviewed the book proposal and provided valuable feedback: Naomi Chedd,

Pamela A. Malone, and Mathew Owen Howard. I am grateful to Al Kaszniak for contributing the Foreword and for continuing to blaze trails connecting Eastern wisdom and Western psychology.

Many students have crossed my path, so I don't want to single any of you out. You are part of my learning, my joy, and my growth. I have come to love you more and more each year. Thank you to the other parts of my community, in particular, the faculty at Sacramento State; "Las Hermanas"; clinical supervisees, Susan Orr, Satsuki Ina, Dave Nylund, Sylvester Bowie, and Dale Russell; as well as Nancy, Liz, and Mike Bein. Nancy, may you have the ultimate journey of wellness and recovery.

I see "the clients" in the office and group rooms, in waiting rooms when I do field visits, in the streets, in respectable jobs, in my dining room, in the university classrooms, in coffee shops, and in community meetings, and I never stop being in awe—thank you for making the world better by being who you are.

About the Author

Andrew Bein, PhD, LCSW, has nearly 30 years of experience as a clinician, consultant, trainer, and researcher. Over the past 15 years he has examined mindfulness applications for therapeutic and direct service contexts, as well as for their utility in enhancing the practitioner's use-of-self. His current book, *Dialectical Behavior Therapy for Wellness and Recovery: Interventions and Activities for Diverse Client Needs*, reflects his DBT-informed group and individual practice conducted in the following settings: dual diagnosis, women with substance abuse, private practice, community mental health, high school, and crisis-residential. He is a full professor with the Division of Social Work at California State University, Sacramento.

Author Index

Subject Index

Self-compassion:
  12-step programs and, 28
  acceptance and, 21
  common humanity and, 27–28, 29
  compassion and, 28–29
  components of, 27–28, 30–31, 32
  cultivation of, 17, 116
  cultural competence and, 33–35
  externalizing mind states and, 32–33
  generating, 151
  intention of, 27–32
  interpersonal skills and, 33
  mindfulness and, 28 (*see also* Mindfulness)
  mindfulness exercises and, 30
  practice model and, xvii
  radical acceptance and, 31–33
  self-kindness and, 27
  situation modification and, 45
  for support, 164, 165
  trauma and, 116
  Wise Mind and, 164
Self-determination, 110
Self-disclosure, practitioner, 146
Self-efficacy, 103
Self-esteem:
  client outcomes and, 134
  cultural competence and, 33–35
  "internalized stigma" and, 66
  self-compassion and, 33
Self-harm:
  emotion regulation and, 65
  as soothing strategy, 51
Self-judgments:
  examples of, 169
  mindfulness and, 35
Self-kindness, 27
Self-Nurturance and Joy, 216–218
Self-observation, 42
Self-reflection, 129
Self-regulation of attention, 36
Self-soothing strategies, 51–52
Serenity Prayer, 49, 50, 210
Shame:
  addiction and, 29
  humiliation and, 120
  pain and, 3
  trauma and, 120
Situation modification:
  example, 44
  mindful approach to, 45
Situation selection, 44
Skillfulness. *See also* Interpersonal skills
  vs. appropriate/inappropriate, 19
  of intention, 21–27
Skills training:
  in DBT-WR model, 11
  emotion regulation and, 119
  task of, 103

Sleeping, trouble with:
  doing what is needed, 204–205
  mindful breaths and, 24–25
"Small mind," "bigger picture" and, 58
Social interactions, emotion regulation and, 18
Social isolation, 66
Societal stigma:
  spirituality and, 65–70
  trauma and, 116
Soothing, 51–52, 177–178
Speech and Telling the Truth, Effective,
    219–222
Spiritual approaches:
  client spirituality, 10–11
  overview, xix
Spirituality:
  expanding the moment and, 62–63
  language and, 143–144
  as liberating force, 63
  as quest/tool, 65–70
  and religion, defined, 63–65
Stigma. *See* Societal stigma
Strengths-oriented language and praise, 34
Stress:
  emotion and, 15
  extreme, 119–121
Stress Reduction Clinic, 138
Strong back, soft front:
  in group setting, 140, 142
  overview of, 130–133
Substance abuse:
  methamphetamine use, 74
  mindfulness and, 42
  overview, xviii
  perinatal drug treatment program, 10
  PTSD and, 93, 113
  self-harm and, 52
  societal stigma and, 66
  spirituality and, 63
  use-of-self and, 139–140
  women and, 93, 113
Substance Abuse and Mental Health Services
    Administration (SAMHSA), 77–78
Substance abuse recovery:
  abstinence and, 78
  DBT-WR and, 106–110
  "dimensions" of, 78
  foundations of, 104–106
  harm reduction and, 110
  meaning of recovery, 77, 78–79
  overview of, 103–104
Suffering to Balance, Finding the Zone: Moving
    From, 212–215
Suicide ideation:
  emotion dysregulation and, 16
  emotions and, 52
  respect for clients and, 95
Survivor shame, 120